Clinical Management of
COVID-19
in India

Clinical Management of
COVID-19
in India

Suresh Kumar MD, FICP

Senior Consultant Physician, Director Professor and Head
Department of Medicine
Maulana Azad Medical College (MAMC) and
Associated LNJP and GB Pant Hospital
New Delhi

Co-authors

Karan Chhabra MD
Senior Resident
Department of Medicine, MAMC
New Delhi

Rajesh Ruttala PhD (Medicine)
Molecular Biologist, MAMC
New Delhi

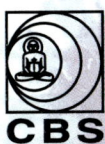

C B S

CBS Publishers & Distributors Pvt Ltd

New Delhi • Bengaluru • Chennai • Kochi • Kolkata • Lucknow • Mumbai
Hyderabad • Jharkhand • Nagpur • Patna • Pune • Uttarakhand

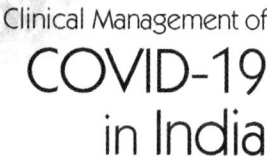

Clinical Management of
COVID-19
in India

ISBN: 978-93-54660-32-0

Copyright © Author and Publisher

First Edition: 2022

Published by Satish Kumar Jain and produced by Varun Jain for

CBS Publishers & Distributors Pvt Ltd
4819/XI Prahlad Street, 24 Ansari Road, Daryaganj, New Delhi 110 002
Ph: 011-23289259, 23266861, 23266867Fax: 011-23243014   Website: www.cbspd.com
e-mail: delhi@cbspd.com; cbspubs@airtelmail.in
Corporate Office: 204 FIE, Industrial Area, Patparganj, Delhi 110 092
Ph: 011-4934 4934   Fax: 011-4934 4935   e-mail: publishing@cbspd.com; publicity@cbspd.com

Branches

- **Bengaluru:** Seema House 2975, 17th Cross, KR Road, Banasankari 2nd Stage, Bengaluru 560 070, Karnataka
  Ph: +91-80-26771678/79   Fax: +91-80-26771680   e-mail: bangalore@cbspd.com
- **Chennai:** 7, Subbaraya Street, Shenoy Nagar, Chennai 600 030, Tamil Nadu
  Ph: +91-44-26260666, 26208620   Fax: +91-44-42032115   e-mail: chennai@cbspd.com
- **Kochi:** 42/1325, 1326, Power House Road, Opp KSEB Power House, Eranakulam 682 018, Kochi, Kerala
  Ph: +91-484-4059061-67   Fax: +91-484-4059065   e-mail: kochi@cbspd.com
- **Kolkata:** 147, Hind Ceramics Compound, 1st Floor, Nilgunj Road, Belghoria, Kolkata-700056, India
  Ph: +91-9096713055/7798394118, 9836841399   e-mail: kolkata@cbspd.com
- **Lucknow:** Basement, Khushnuma Complex, 7 Meerabai Marg (Behind Jawahar Bhawan), Lucknow-226001, UP, India
  Ph: +0522-4000032   e-mail: tiwari.lucknow@cbspd.com
- **Mumbai:** PWD Shed, Gala no 25/26, Ramchandra Bhatt Marg, Next to JJ Hospital Gate no. 2, Opp. Union Bank of India, Noorbaug, Mumbai-400009, Maharashtra
  Ph: +91-22-66661880/89   e-mail: mumbai@cbspd.com

Representatives

• **Hyderabad**	0-9885175004	• **Jharkhand**	0-9811541605	• **Nagpur**	0-9421945513
• **Patna**	0-9334159340	• **Pune**	0-9623451994	• **Uttarakhand**	0-9716462459

Printed at: Goyal Offset Works Pvt. Ltd.

Contributors

Anil Chokan
Senior Consultant Radiologist
New Delhi

Anju Garg
Director Professor and Head
Radiodiagnosis
MAMC, New Delhi

Ashad Narayanan
Resident, LNH
New Delhi

Asmita M Rathore
Director Professor and Head
Obs and Gynae
MAMC, New Delhi

Ekta Gupta
Additional Professor
Department of Virology, ILBS
Vasant Kunj, Delhi

Farah Husain
Specialist, Anaesthesiology and Intensive Care
MAMC, New Delhi

Gunjan Manchanda
Specialist, Anaesthesiology and Intensive Care
MAMC, New Delhi

Harpreet Singh
Associate Professor, Medicine
MAMC, New Delhi

Himansu Sekhar Mahapatra
Professor and Head
Nephrology, RML Hospital
New Delhi

Karan Chhabra
Senior Resident Medicine
MAMC, New Delhi

Kartik Singhai
SR Psychiatry
AIIMS, Jodhpur, Rajasthan

Krishna Agarwal
Professor
Obs and Gynae
MAMC, New Delhi

Lalita Chaudhary
Director Professor
Anaesthesia
MAMC, New Delhi

Lovenish Bains
Surgeon
MAMC, New Delhi

Mohit D. Gupta
Professor Cardiology
GB Pant Hospital, New Delhi

Munisha Agarwal
Director Professor and Head
Anaesthesiology and Intensive Care
MAMC, New Delhi

Nandini Sharma
Director Professor
PSM MAMC
New Delhi

Niharika Dhiman
Associate Professor
Obs and Gynae
MAMC, New Delhi

Pradeep Kumar
Associate Professor Medicine
MAMC, New Delhi

Rajdeep Singh
Professor, Surgery
MAMC, New Delhi

Rajesh Ruttala
Consultant/Molecular Biologist
LNH, New Delhi

Sandeep Garg
Director Professor, Medicine
MAMC, New Delhi

SK Sarin
Director, ILBS (Padma Bhushan Awardee)
Vasant Kunj, New Delhi

Sunita Aggarwal
Director Professor, Medicine
MAMC, New Delhi

Urmila Jhamb
Director Professor, Paediatrics
MAMC, New Delhi

Vandana Saith
Specialist, Anaesthesiology and Intensive Care
MAMC, New Delhi

Vikas Manchanda
Professor, Microbiology
MAMC, New Delhi

Foreword

Coronavirus disease 2019 (COVID-19) (severe acute respiratory syndrome coronavirus 2 [SARS-CoV-2]) is a global health and economic crisis. This pandemic has affected over 215 countries around the world with 19.1 Cr cases (as on July 20, 2021) globally with more than 41 lakh deaths, and the number is increasing rapidly.

This is a great challenge for healthcare providers of India as there is a substantial risk to the life of doctors and healthcare workers because of this deadly virus. Advances in medical sciences have been spectacular, but at the same time, newer viruses, like Ebola, Hantavirus and SARS-CoV-2 have posed new challenges to the existence of mankind.

In India, molecular diagnostics RT-PCR labs are limited in number for diagnosis of all suspected cases. Social distancing, quarantine and isolation, active tracing of contacts of suspected and treatment of confirmed cases are at war footing in India. This has been very successful so far for breaking the chain of viral transmission.

We are greatly successful in containing the virus so far and limiting the number of deaths in India.

Rapidly expanding genetic knowledge and antiviral drugs have made significant improvement in HIV and HCV treatment. We hope, new treatment will soon be available of COVID-19 patients also.

This book has been developed with a comprehensive and analytic approach with excellent flowcharts for day-to-day management of COVID-19 patients.

This will be very useful for physicians, researchers and healthcare workers. All the best for great work of Prof Suresh Kumar and his team for the highly incredible job they have done in such a short period.

SK Sarin
Director
Institute of Liver and Biliary Sciences
New Delhi

Preface

We decided to write a medical book about the ongoing SARS-COV-2 pandemic, presenting the scientific data and up-to-date literature for the fellow physician community and a guide for residents doing COVID duties. A scientific book presents "plenty of information", however, when we became aware of the new coronavirus epidemic in mid-January 2020, we immediately felt that time had come to bring out a textbook from the largest COVID dedicated centre in NCT of Delhi fulfilling the purpose.

People all over the world will have to adapt and invent new lifestyles in what has been the most disruptive event since World War II. Imposing and enforcing strict quarantine measures and isolating millions of people might have seemed a distant possibility before the year 2020, but is now a reality in many countries.

We believe that the current situation needs a new type of textbook with continuous updates. Humanity is confronting an unknown and threatening disease which is often severe and fatal. Healthcare systems are overwhelmed and the treating physicians need clear understanding and concepts to provide optimal standard of care.

We believe a clear head is crucial in times of over-information, with dozens of scientific papers and research published everyday, news about hundreds of studies being planned or already on the way and social media blending hard data with rumors and unverified news. The tedious work of screening the scientific literature and the scientific data has to be done—regularly and constantly, like a Swiss watch. The proposed book covers relevant chapters from apex faculty who are masters in their respective fields from the premier teaching institutes in India.

Suresh Kumar

Contents

Epidemiology

Nandini Sharma

- It was in late December 2019 that a cluster of patients was admitted to hospitals with the initial diagnosis of pneumonia of unknown etiology. These patients were found to have an epidemiological link to a seafood and wet animal wholesale market in Wuhan, Hubei Province, China.
- Between December 18, 2019 and December 29, 2019, 5 patients were hospitalized with acute respiratory distress syndrome (ARDS) and one of them died. By January 2, 2020, 41 patients admitted to the hospital had been identified as having laboratory-confirmed coronavirus disease 2019 (COVID-19) infection. Less than-half of these patients had underlying diseases, including diabetes, hypertension and cardio-vascular disease. This disease, caused by severe acute respiratory syndrome corona-virus 2 (SARS-CoV-2), was named COVID-19 on January 12, 2020.
- As of January 22, 2020, 571 cases of COVID-19 were reported in 25 provinces in China. As of January 30, 2020, 7734 cases were confirmed in China and 90 others were reported from other countries including Taiwan, Thailand, Vietnam, Malaysia, Nepal, Sri Lanka, Cambodia, Japan, Singapore, Republic of Korea, United Arab Emirates, United States, The Philippines, India, Australia, Canada, Finland, France and Germany. The case fatality rate was estimated as 2.2%.
- Currently, over 220 countries have reported confirmed case of COVID-19 with a total of above 188 million cases with more than 40 lakh fatalities (as on July 14, 2021). India has reported around 30.9 million cases till now including 4,11,615 deaths. (July 14, 2021).
- World Health Organization (WHO) declared COVID-19 as Public Health Emergency of International Concern (PHEIC) on 30th of January, 2020. Since then, the world has seen unprecedented measures to curb the spread of infection, such as nation wide lockdowns.
- The median R, (reproductive number which refers to the average number of individuals infected by an index case) is between 2 and 2.5 for the current pandemic. This estimated R is less than the previous SARS-CoV epidemic in 2002–2003 which was approximately 3.
- Data from the first cases in Wuhan and investigations from the China CDC (center for disease control and prevention) and local CDCs suggest that the incubation time could be usually within 3 to 7 days and up to 2 weeks, as the longest time from infection to symptom onset has been noted to be 12.5 days [95% confidence interval (CI), 9.2–18].

TRANSMISSION

- The initial cases of COVID-19 were linked to direct exposure to the Huanan Seafood Wholesale Market of Wuhan; hence, animal-to-human transmission was considered as the main mechanism. Later cases were; however, not associated with this exposure mechanism. Therefore, it was concluded that human-to-human transmission is also possible, and symptomatic people most frequently had spread the infection.
- The possibility of transmission before symptom onset seems to be infrequent, yet it cannot be completely excluded. Additionally, there are suggestions that asymptomatic individuals could transmit the virus.
- Use of isolation thus seems the best way to contain this epidemic.
- SARS-CoV-2 RNA has also been detected in blood and stool specimens. Live virus has been cultured from stool in some cases, but according to a joint WHO-China report, fecal-oral transmission did not appear to be a significant factor in infection spread.

MODES OF TRANSMISSION OF VIRUS CAUSING COVID-19

- Current evidence indicates that the virus causing COVID-19 is transmitted among people through respiratory droplets and contact routes.
- Droplet transmission occurs when a person is in close contact, i.e. within 1 m, with someone having respiratory symptoms (e.g. coughing or sneezing) and therefore, there is a risk that his/her mucosae (mouth and nose) or conjunctiva (eyes) are exposed to potentially infective respiratory droplets (which are generally considered to be >5–10 m in diameter).
- Transmission could also occur through fomites in the immediate environment around the infected person.
- Transmission of the COVID-19 virus can, therefore, occur by direct contact with infected people and indirect contact with surfaces in the immediate environment or with objects used on the infected person, such as stethoscope or thermometer.
- Airborne transmission differs from droplet transmission as it refers to the presence of microbes within droplet nuclei, which are generally considered as particles <5 μm in diameter, and which result from the evaporation of larger droplets or exist within dust particles. They may remain in the air for long periods of time and can be transmitted to others overdistances >1 m.
- Airborne transmission of COVID-19 virus may occur in specific circumstances in which certain procedures that generate aerosols are performed (such as endotracheal intubation, bronchoscopy, open suctioning, administration of nebulized treatment, manual ventilation before intubation, turning the patient to the prone position, disconnecting the patient from the ventilator, noninvasive positive-pressure ventilation, tracheostomy and cardiopulmonary resuscitation).
- In an analysis of 75,465 COVID-19 cases in China, airborne transmission was not reported. There is evidence that COVID-19 infection may cause intestinal infection and be present in faeces. However, only one study till date has cultured the COVID-19 virus from a single stool specimen.

There are no reports of feco-oral transmission of the COVID-19 virus thus far. As, the outbreak continues to evolve, new things are being learnt about this new virus everyday. Summarized below are the facts reported about transmission of the COVID-19 virus. Additionally, it provides a brief overview of available evidence on transmission from symptomatic, presymptomatic and asymptomatic people infected with COVID-19.

Symptomatic Transmission

- A symptomatic COVID-19 case is one who has developed signs and symptoms consistent with COVID-19 infection. Symptomatic transmission is the transmission from a person while they have symptoms.
- Epidemiology and virologic studies have shown that COVID-19 is largely transmitted from symptomatic people to others who come in dose contact by means of respiratory droplets, direct contact with infected persons or through contact with contaminated objects and surfaces.
- Data from clinical and virologic studies that assessed repeated biological samples from confirmed patients suggest that SARS-CoV-2 shedding is highest in upper respiratory tract (nose and throat) early in the course of the disease. This means within the first 3 days from onset of symptoms.

Presymptomatic Transmission

- The incubation period for COVID-19, i.e. the time from exposure to the virus to symptom onset, is an average of 5–6 days, but it can be up to 14 days. During this period, which is also known as the "presymptomatic" period, some infected persons can be contagious. Therefore, transmission from a presymptomatic individual can occur prior to symptom onset.
- Some case reports and studies have shown presymptomatic transmission through contact tracing efforts and investigation of clusters of confirmed cases. Data suggest that some people can test positive for COVID-19 from 1 to 3 days before developing symptoms.
- It seems possible that people infected with COVID-19 could transmit the virus before the onset of significant symptoms. However, presymptomatic transmission still requires the virus to be spread through infectious droplets or through touching contaminated surfaces.

Asymptomatic Transmission

- A person who is infected with COVID-19 but does not develop symptoms is an asymptomatic laboratory-confirmed case.
- As per a recent study, the viral load detected in asymptomatic populations was similar to that in symptomatic patients, indicating that asymptomatic infections have the potential for transmission, which may occur early in the course of infection.

SARS-CoV-2 Variants

Since December 2020 many variants of SARS-CoV-2 has been identified as seen with other SARS coronaviruses. WHO has identified these variants as variants of interest (VOI), variants of concern (VOCs) and variants of high consequences. These variants can be highly transmissible and change the course of COVID-19 epidemiology and result in potential public health intervention measures to fail. Currently, WHO has designated the variants of concern with Greek letters Alpha (first identified in UK), Beta (First identified in South Africa), Gamma (First identified in Brazil) and Delta (first identified in India in May 2021).

HOST FACTORS

Although SARS-CoV-2 can infect people of all ages, the following groups are more vulnerable and are likely to develop more serious disease:
- Elderly (age >60 years)
- Diabetes
- Hypertension
- Pre-existing heart disease
- Immunodeficiency
- Healthcare workers
- Pre-existing pulmonary disease
- Economic inequality.

ENVIRONMENTAL FACTORS

Factors that enhance transmission of the disease are:
- Overcrowding
- Mass gathering.

PREVENTIVE MEASURES

- Vaccination
- Restricting international travel
- Social distancing
- Avoiding mass gatherings
- Regular handwashing/using hand sanitizers
- National/state level lockdowns.

BIBLIOGRAPHY

1. Available at: www.worldometer.info/coronavirus.
2. Bauch CT, Lloyd-Smith JO, Coffee MP, et al. Dynamically modeling SARS and other newly emerging respiratory illnesses: past, present, and future. Epidemiology. 2005; 16(6):791–801.
3. Li Q, Guan X, Wu P, et al. Early transmission dynamics in Wuhan, China, of novel coronavirus-infected pneumonia. N Engl J Med. 2020;382(13):1199–2007.
4. Liu J, Liao X, Qian S, et al. Community transmission of severe acute respiratory syndrome coronavirus 2, Shenzhen, China, 2020. Emerg Infect Dis. 2020;26(6):1320–3.
5. Ong SWX, Tan YK, Chia PY, et al. Air, surface environmental, and personal protective equipment contamination by severe acute respiratory syndrome coronavirus 2 (SARSCoV-2) from a symptomatic patient. JAMA. 2020;323(16):1610–2.
6. Ren LL, Wang YM, Wu ZQ, et al. Identification of a novel corona virus causing severe pneumonia in human: a descriptive study. Chin Med J (Engl). 2020; 133(9):1015–24.
7. Tracking SARS-CoV-2 variants (who.int).

8. W~lfelR, Corman VM, Guggemos W, et al. Virological assessment of hospitalized patients with COVID-2019. Nature. 2020;581(7809):465–9.

9. Wang W, Xu Y, Gao R, et al. Detection of SARS-CoV-2 in different types of clinical specimens. JAMA. 2020;323(18):1843–4.

10. Wei WE, Li Z, Chiew CJ, et al. Presymptomatic transmission of SARS-CoV-2- Singapore, January 23-March 16, 2020. MMWR Morb Mortal Wkly Rep. 2020;69:411–5.

11. World Health Organization. Report of the WHO-China Joint Mission on Coronavirus Disease 2019 (COVID-19). 16-24 February, 2020 [Internet]. Geneva: World Health Organization; 2020. Available at: https://www.who. int/docs/default-source/coronaviruse/who-china-joint-mission-on-covid19-finalreport.pdf

12. Zhang Y, Chen C, Zhu S, et al. Isolation of 2019-nCoV from a stool specimen of a laboratory-confirmed case of the coronavirus disease 2019 (COVID-19). China CDC Weekly. 2020;2(8):123–4.

13. Zou L, Ruan F, Huang M, et al. SARS-CoV-2 viral load in upper respiratory specimens of infected patients. N Engl J Med. 2020;382(12):1177–9.

Virology

Rajesh Ruttala, Ashad Narayanan

INTRODUCTION

Coronavirus comprises of a large family of viruses that are common in human beings as well as animals, such as camels, cattle, cats and bats. Seven different strains of coronaviruses have been identified that infect humans (Fig. 2.1).

a. 229E (alpha coronavirus)

b. NL63 (alpha coronavirus)

c. OC43 (beta coronavirus)

d. HKU1 (beta coronavirus)

e. MERS-CoV (beta coronavirus that causes middle east respiratory syndrome or MERS)

f. SARS-CoV (beta coronavirus that causes severe acute respiratory syndrome or SARS)

g. SARS-CoV-2 (the novel coronavirus that causes COVID-19)

SARS and MERS are caused by coronaviruses that jumped from animals to humans. Over 8,000 individuals were infected by SARS, and nearly 800 died of the illness (mortality rate of approximately 10%), before it was brought under control in 2003. MERS continues to resurge in sporadic cases. Overall, 2,465 laboratory-confirmed cases of MERS have been reported since 2012, with 850 deaths (mortality rate of 34.5%).

- The virus that causes COVID-19 is designated as SARS-CoV-2; previously, referred to as 2019-nCoV.
- Towards the end of December 2019, this novel coronavirus was identified as a cause of upper and lower respiratory tract infections in Wuhan, Hubei Province, China. It spread at a rapid pace, leading to an epidemic across China and then gradually spread to other parts of the world in pandemic proportions. It has affected almost every continent, except Antarctica.
- In February 2020, the WHO designated the disease COVID-19, which stands for coronavirus disease 2019.

VIROLOGY

- Coronaviruses are enveloped viruses with a positive sense single-stranded RNA genome. Four coronavirus genera—α, β, γ, δ—have been identified thus far.

- In late December 2019, patients having cough, fever and dyspnea with ARDS due to an unidentified microbial infection were reported in Wuhan, China.
- Virus genome sequencing of 5 patients with pneumonia hospitalized between December 18 and December 29, 2019, pointed to the presence of a previously unknown β-CoV strain.
- This novel β-CoV was given the name "SARS-CoV-2" by the International Virus Classification Commission. The virus has round or elliptic and pleomorphic form, with a diameter of around 60–140 nm.
- Like other coronaviruses, it appears to be sensitive to ultraviolet rays and heat.

AGENTS USED IN INACTIVATING COVID-19

Lipid solvents including:

- Ether (75%)
- Ethanol
- Chlorine-containing disinfectant
- Peroxyacetic acid
- Chloroform, except for chlorhexidine.

VIRAL GENOME

- The SARS-CoV-2 genome is similar to that of typical coronaviruses and comprises of nearly 10 open reading frames (ORFs).
- The first ORFs (ORF1a/b) on nearly two-thirds of viral RNA are translated into two large polyproteins.
- In SARS-CoV and MERS-CoV, two polyproteins (pp1a and pp1ab) get processed to 16 nonstructural proteins (nsp1–nsp16), giving rise to the viral replicase transcriptase complex.
- The nsps rearrange the membranes that originate from the rough endoplasmic reticulum (RER) into double-membrane vesicles, where viral replication and transcription are known to occur.
- The other ORFs on the one-third of the genome encode four key structural proteins namely spike (S), envelope (E), nucleocapsid (N) and membrane (M) proteins. Additionally, there are several accessory proteins with unknown functions, which do not have a role in viral replication.
- These genomic analyses suggest that SARS-CoV-2 has possibly evolved from a strain found in bats.
- The potential amplifying mammalian host, which is an intermediate between bats and humans is; however, not clearly known, although some have suggested pangolins to be the intermediate host. The mutation in the original strain could have directly incited virulence towards humans. Hence, it is not confirmed that this intermediary exists.

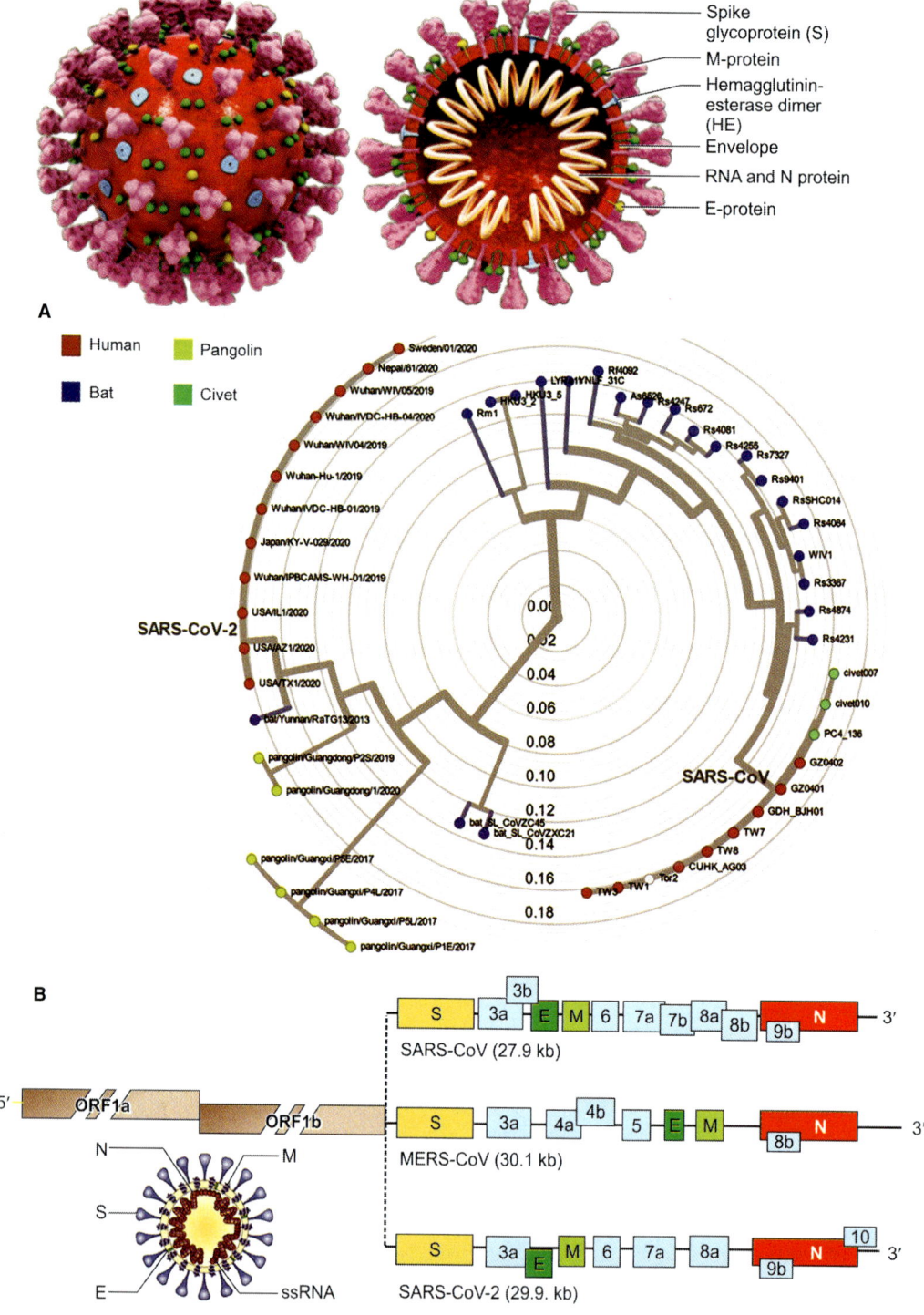

Fig. 2.1: Phylogenetic tree of SARS-like coronaviruses complete genome sequences and genome of SARS-CoV, MERS-CoV and SARS CoV-2 (*Source:* Li X, Geng M, Peng Y, Meng L, Lu S. Molecular immune pathogenesis and diagnosis of COVID-19. *J Pharm Anal.* 2020;10(2):102–108.)

CORONAVIRUS REPLICATION AND PATHOGENESIS

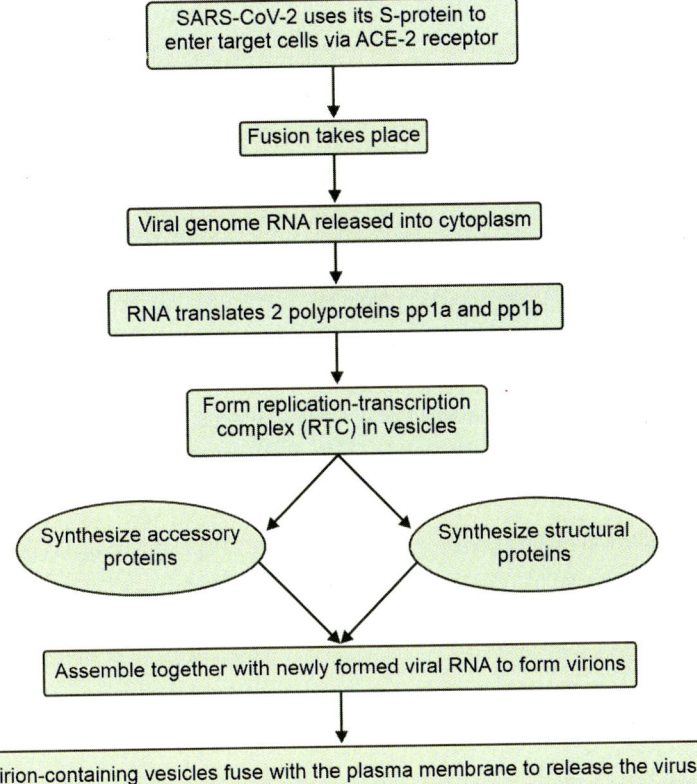

Pathogenesis

Suresh Kumar, Karan Chhabra

- After entering the cells, viral antigens are presented by the APCs (antigen presenting cells). The antigen presentation of SARS-CoV mainly depends on major histo-compatibility complex (MHC) class I molecules (Fig. 3.1).

Human leukocyte antigen (HLA) polymorphisms with susceptibility to SARS-CoV	HLA polymorphisms protective for SARS-CoV
• HLA-B*4601	• HLA-DR0301
• HLA-B*0703	• HLA-Cw1502
• HLA-DRB1*1202	• HLA-A*0201
• HLA-Cw*0801	

- Moreover, gene polymorphisms of mannose-binding lectin (MBL) associated with antigen presentation are also associated with the risk of SARS-CoV infection.
- Similar researches pertaining specifically to SARS-CoV-2 will provide valuable information for prevention, treatment and mechanism of COVID-19.

ROLE OF IMMUNITY AND CYTOKINE STORM

- Recent studies have shown that there is a reduction in the number of CD4+ and CD8+ T cells.
- The main cause of mortality in COVID-19 infection is ARDS. One of the key mechanisms behind ARDS is cytokine storm, which is the fatal uncontrolled systemic inflammatory response that occurs as a result of the release of large amounts of pro-inflammatory cytokines including interleukin [IL]-1β, IL-6, IL-12, IL-18, IL-33, interferon [IFN] α and γ, tumor necrosis factor [TNF] β and TGFβ.
- The cytokine storm incites a violent attack by the immune system to the body, causing ARDS and multiple organ failure, and finally resulting in death in severe cases of SARS-CoV-2 infection; the same is seen in SARS-CoV and MERS-CoV infection (Fig. 3.2).

IMMUNE EVASION BY CORONAVIRUS

- To better survive in host cells, SARS-CoV and MERS-CoV use multiple strategies to avoid immune responses.

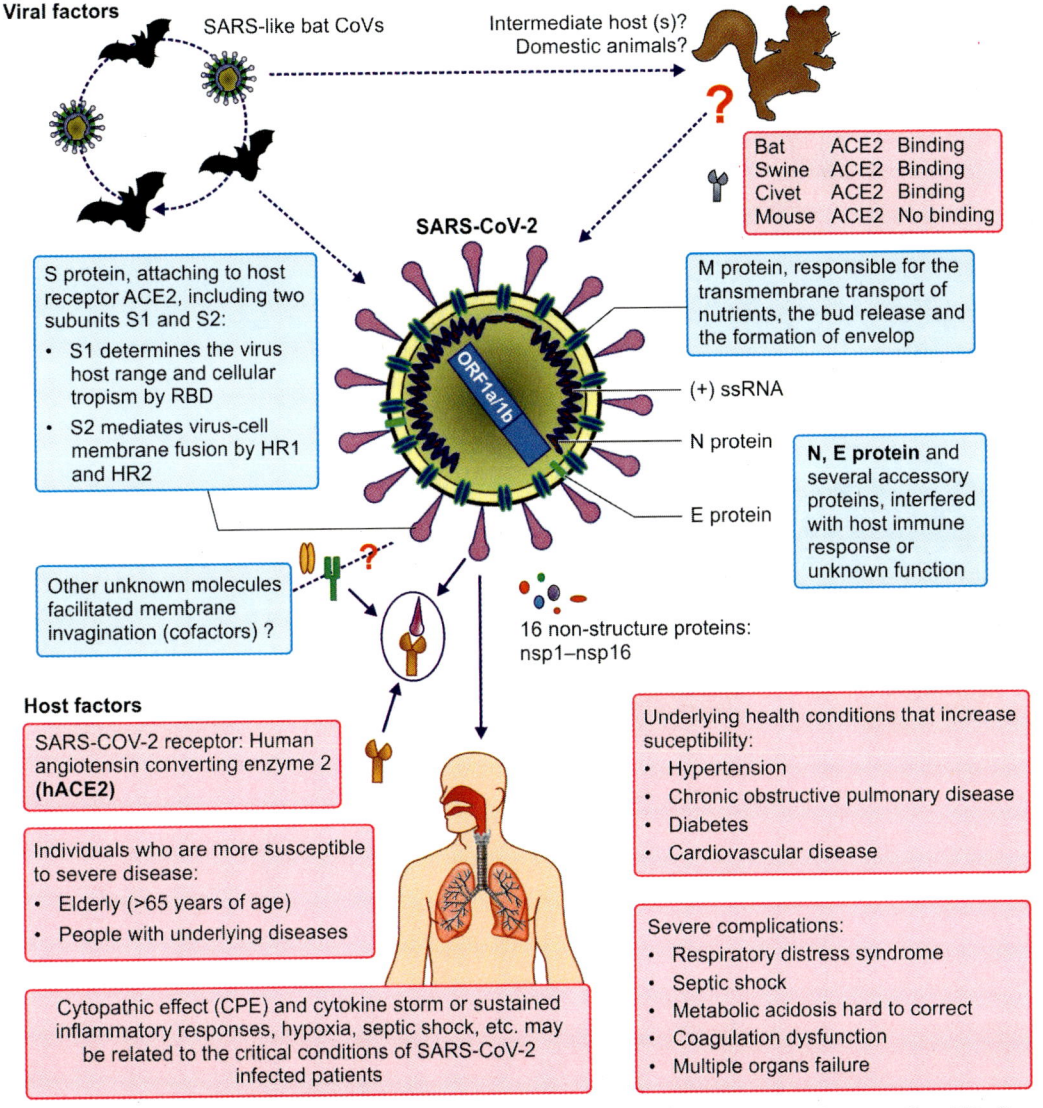

Fig. 3.1: Viral and host factors that influence the pathogenesis of SARS-CoV-2 (*Source:* Guo YR, Cao QD, Hong ZS, et al. The origin, transmission and clinical therapies on coronavirus disease 2019 (COVID-19) outbreak—an update on the status. Mil Med Res. 2020;7(1):11.)

- The evolutionarily conserved microbial structures called pathogen-associated molecular patterns (PAMPs) can be recognized by pattern recognition receptors (PRRs).
- However, SARS-CoV and MERS-CoV can induce the production of double-membrane vesicles that lack PRRs and then replicate in these vesicles, thereby avoiding the host detection of their dsRNA.

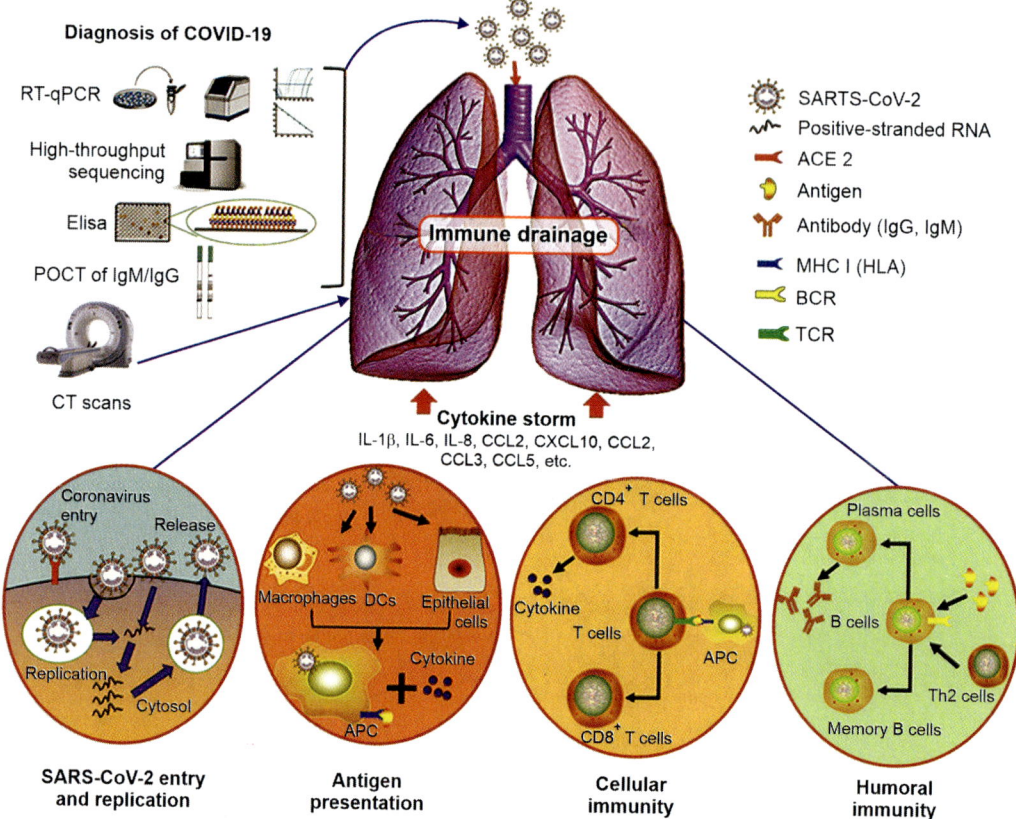

Fig. 3.2: Cytokine storm in COVID-19 infection *(Source:* Li X, Geng M, Peng Y, Meng L, Lu S. Molecular immune pathogenesis and diagnosis of COVID-19. *J Pharm Anal.* 2020;10(2):102–108.)

Clinical Features

Suresh Kumar, Neeraj Azad Yadav, Anil Chokan

Incubation period: While the exact incubation period is not known, it is generally considered to be between 2 and 14 days following exposure, with most cases seen within 5 days after exposure.

Illness severity: Most cases are self-limiting. More severe illness is seen in the elderly or in patients with underlying medical conditions. According to a report from Chinese CDC that involved nearly 44,500 confirmed cases, **mild illness** was observed in 81% patients; **Severe illness,** i.e. hypoxemia, >50% lung involvement on imaging within 24–48 hours, was reported in 14%; **Critical disease** (respiratory failure, shock, multi-organ dysfunction syndrome) was evident in 5%. Overall **case fatality rate** was estimated as 2.3–5%.

Age affected: It mostly affects middle-aged (>30 years) and elderly. Symptomatic infection in children has been uncommon, and when it occurred, it was usually mild.

Clinical Presentation

A study with 1,099 patients with COVID-19 pneumonia in Wuhan revealed that the most common clinical features at the onset of illness were:

- Fever (88%)
- Fatigue (38%)
- Dry cough (67%)
- Myalgias (14.9%)
- Dyspnea (18.7%)

Pneumonia seems to be the most common and severe manifestation of infection. In these patients, breathing difficulty developed after a median of 5 days of illness. ARDS was noted in 3.4% of patients.

Other symptoms include: Headache, sore throat, rhinorrhea, and gastrointestinal symptoms.

RISK FACTORS FOR SEVERE ILLNESS

Severe illness can be noted in otherwise healthy individuals of any age. However, it usually occurs in adults with advanced age or underlying medical comorbidities. Comorbidities linked with severe illness and mortality include:

- Cardiovascular disease
- Diabetes mellitus
- Hypertension
- Chronic lung disease
- Cancer
- Chronic kidney disease.

The United States Centers for Disease Control and Prevention (CDC) also includes immunocompromising conditions, severe obesity [body mass index (BMI) ≥40], and liver disease as potential risk factors for severe illness.

Laboratory features that have been associated with worse outcomes include:
- Lymphopenia
- Deranged kidney function test (KFT) and liver function test (LFT)
- Raised creatine phosphokinase (CPK)/troponin
- Prolonged prothrombin time (PT); raised D-dimer
- High lactate dehydrogenase (LDH) levels
- Raised C-reactive protein (CRP)/ferritin levels.

LABORATORY FINDINGS

White Blood Cell Count

- White blood cell (WBC) count can vary and does not provide accurate information regarding COVID-19.
- Leukopenia, leukocytosis and lymphopenia have been reported.
- Lymphopenia is more common, and is evident in over 80% of patients.
- Mild thrombocytopenia is usually seen. However, thrombocytopenia is a poor prognostic sign.

INFLAMMATORY MARKERS

Serum Procalcitonin

Serum procalcitonin is usually normal at admission; however, it tends to increases in patients requiring ICU care. A study revealed that high D-dimer and lymphopenia were associated with poor prognosis.

C-reactive Protein

CRP is increased in COVID-19 infection. This seems to track with disease severity and prognosis.

In patients with severe respiratory failure with a normal CRP level, an alternative diagnosis should always be looked for.

Laboratory Diagnosis of COVID-19 Infection

Ekta Gupta, Abhishek Padhi, Shiv Kumar Sarin

BACKGROUND

Coronavirus disease 2019 (COVID-19) is an infection caused by the novel coronavirus SARS-CoV-2. SARS-CoV-2 is a member of the subgenus *Sarbecovirus* (beta-CoV lineage B) of the broad family *Coronaviridae.* They are enveloped and have a nonsegmented, single-stranded, positive-sense ribonucleic acid (ssRNA+) as their nuclear material. The disease spectrum ranges from mild asymptomatic cases to severe acute respiratory illness (SARI). Early diagnosis is the key for prompt management of cases and control of the spread of the virus. Hence, laboratory diagnosis of SARS-CoV-2 holds the key in containing and restricting the COVID-19 pandemic.

SPECIMEN

COVID-19 primarily causes acute respiratory illness, so the primary samples to be collected are those from the respiratory tract.

a. **Upper respiratory samples:** Oropharyngeal and nasopharyngeal swabs (Dacron or polyester flocked swabs) should be collected properly from the proper anatomical sites and placed in a single viral transport media (VTM) tube to increase the viral load.

b. **Lower respiratory samples:** In patients with more severe respiratory disease, sputum, endotracheal aspirate or bronchoalveolar lavage may be collected.

Other samples that may be collected are:
- Paired Sera (acute and convalescent)—for detection of antibodies against SARS-CoV-2
- Lung tissue—for postmortem study
- Blood—collected from all positive cases
- Stool—research has shown evidence of gastrointestinal infection by SARS-CoV-2.

After the samples are collected, they should be properly labeled and packed following the triple packaging method (Fig. 5.1) and should be transported to the nearest laboratory maintaining adequate cold chain. If the samples are to be processed within 5 days, they can be stored at a temperature of 4°C and if a delay of more than 5 days is expected, they have to be stored at a temperature of –77°C.

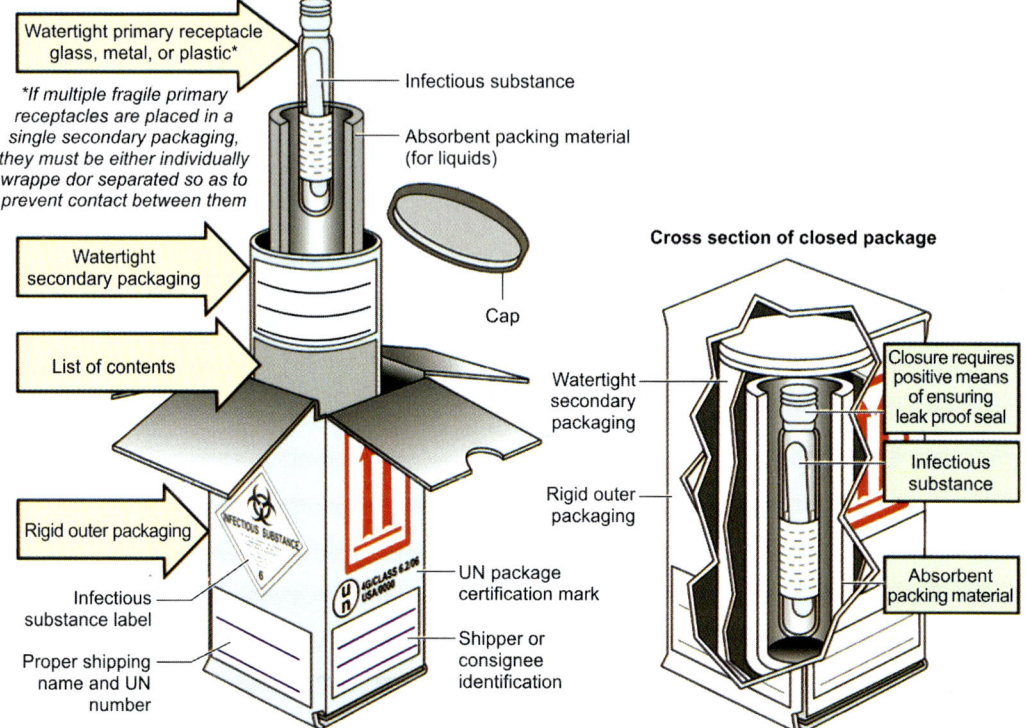

Watertight primary receptacle glass, metal, or plastic*

*If multiple fragile primary receptacles are placed in a single secondary packaging, they must be either individually wrappe dor separated so as to prevent contact between them

Infectious substance

Absorbent packing material (for liquids)

Watertight secondary packaging

Cap

List of contents

Rigid outer packaging

Infectious substance label

Proper shipping name and UN number

UN package certification mark

Shipper or consignee identification

Cross section of closed package

Watertight secondary packaging

Rigid outer packaging

Closure requires positive means of ensuring leak proof seal

Infectious substance

Absorbent packing material

Fig. 5.1: Triple packing of specimen (3 packaging). (*Source:* Packaging and Shipping Clinical Specimens Diagram | For Laboratory Personnel. Ebola (Ebola Virus Disease). CDC. Available at: https://www.cdc.gov/vhf/ebola/laboratory-personnel/shipping-specimens.html)

Testing strategy varies among different countries depending on the stage at which the pandemic is in that specific country. In India, the Ministry of Health and Family Welfare (MoHFW), through the Indian Council of Medical Research (ICMR), keeps updating the testing strategy time to time. Following is the criteria of "WHOM TO TEST" in India:

1. All symptomatic individuals who have undertaken international travel in the last 14 days.
2. All symptomatic contacts of laboratory confirmed cases.
3. All symptomatic healthcare workers.
4. All patients with SARI (fever and cough and/or shortness of breath).
5. Asymptomatic direct and high-risk contacts of a confirmed case should be tested once between day 5 and day 14 of coming in his/her contact.
6. In hotspots/cluster and in large migration gatherings/evacuees centers
7. All symptomatic influenza like illness (fever, cough, sore throat, runny nose)
   a. Within 7 days of illness: Real-time reverse transcriptase polymerase chain reaction (rRT-PCR)
   b. After 7 days of illness: Antibody test (if negative, confirmed by rRT-PCR).

Biosafety Precautions for Handling COVID-19 Specimens
- Healthcare professional collecting samples from suspected patients should don proper personal protective equipment (PPE).
- Sample processing and PCR assay can be done in a biosafety level-2 (bsl-2) facility but biosafety level-3 (bsl-3) precautions should be followed by healthcare workers.

LABORATORY TESTING OF COVID-19

Timely diagnosis of COVID-19 is important for the management of the disease and breaking the chain of transmission of SARS-CoV-2. Following are the various modalities by which detection of SARS-CoV-2 is possible:
- Nucleic acid amplification testing (NAAT)
- Sequencing
- Serological assays
- Viral culture.

Nucleic Acid Amplification Testing

Confirmation of cases of COVID-19 is based on the detection of viral RNA by NAAT such as real-time reverse transcriptase polymerase chain reactions (RT-qPCR) (Fig. 5.2). Various genes of the viral genome are targeted in the PCR reaction.

Molecular targets used for PCR assays:
- Structural genes:
  - Envelope glycoprotein spike (S)
  - Envelope (E)
  - Transmembrane (M)
  - Helicase (Hel)
  - Nucleocapsid (N)
- Species specific accessory genes:
  - RNA-dependent RNA polymerase (RdRp)
  - Hemagglutinin-esterase (HE)
  - Open reading frames ORF1a and ORF1b

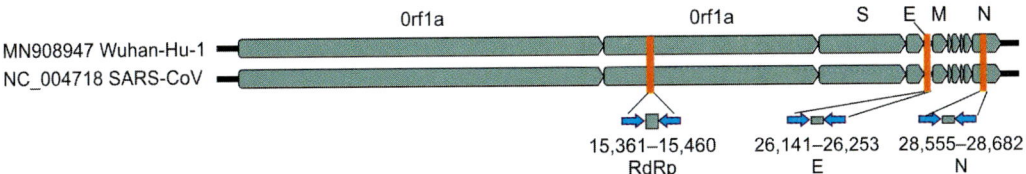

Fig. 5.2: Relative positions of amplicon targets on SARS-CoV-2 genome

ORF: Open reading frame; RdRp: RNA dependent RNA polymerase; E: Envelope protein gene; N: Nucleocapsid protein gene; M: Membrane protein gene; S: Spike protein gene.
Numbers below amplicons are genome positions according to SARS-CoV, GenBank NC_004718.
(*Source:* Corman et al. Detection of 2019 novel coronavirus (2019-nCoV) by real-time RT-PCR . Euro Surveill. 2020 Jan 23; 25(3): 2000045)

WHO recommends that at least two genes should be detected for the diagnosis of COVID-19):
- Screening assay (*Example:* E gene assay)
- Confirmatory assay (*Example:* RdRp assay).

Reporting of PCR assays:
- Qualitative PCR test
- Fluorescence is detected against a gene
- The point at which the fluorescence starts is the cycle threshold (Ct) of the run
- A minimum of 45 cycles are run for a PCR assay
- A sample is considered as positive when both screening as well as confirmatory genes are detected with a Ct value ≤38–40 for both screening as well as for the confirmatory assay.

The rate of positivity of PCR assay varies with specimen used for testing. PCR assay positivity rate for various samples used is given below.

Sample used	Rate of positivity (%)
Bronchoalveolar lavage fluid	93
Sputum	72
Nasal swab	63
Fibrobronchoscope biopsy	46
Pharyngeal swabs	32
Feces	29
Blood	1

Commercial kits

Many commercial kits have been approved by the US Food and Drug Administration (FDA) on the Emergency Use Authorization (EUA) basis to expedite the kit availability. Below is the list of diagnostic kits approved by the ICMR along with their targets.

Name of company	Name of the kit	Gene target
Altona diagnostics	RealStar SARS-CoV-2 RT-PCR Kit 1.0	Lineage B-beta CoV (E gene) SARS-CoV-2 (S gene)
ABI	TaqMan 2019-nCoV Control Kit v1	SARS-CoV-2: ORF1ab gene S gene N gene
Roche	LightMix Modular SARS and Wuhan CoV E-gene	76 bp E gene (SARS-CoV, SARS-CoV-2 and bat SARS viruses)
Roche	LightMix Modular SARS and Wuhan CoV N gene	126 bp N gene (SARS-CoV, SARS-CoV-2 and bat SARS viruses)
Roche	LightMix Modular Wuhan RdRp gene	100 bp RdRp gene (SARS-CoV, SARS-CoV-2 and bat SARS viruses)
Seegene	Allplex 2019-nCoV assay	Sarbecoviruses (E gene) SARS-CoV-2 (RdRp and N genes)
SD Biosensor	nCoV Real-Time Detection Kit	SARS-CoV-2 (RdRp and E genes)

Near point of care molecular assays
- Because the extraction protocol requires bsl-3 facility, is labor intensive and time consuming, the need of the hour is to reduce the duration of the PCR assay, a cartridge-based near point of care molecular assay.
- These are cartridge-based self-enclosed systems integrating nucleic acid extraction, amplification and detection.
- Results are quick and can be used as point of care test with minimal requirement of biosafety precautions.

Other molecular methods like loop-mediated isothermal amplification, multiplex isothermal amplification, microarray detection, *clustered regularly interspaced short palindromic repeats (CRISPR)*-based assays are being developed and evaluated globally for the diagnosis of COVID-19.

Sequencing
- Not used routinely for the diagnosis of SARS-CoV-2.
- Sequencing methods played a major role in the initial identification of SARS-CoV-2.
- Next generation sequencing and metagenomic next generation sequencing will be needed for determining mutations in the genome of SARS-CoV-2.

Serological Assay
- Serological assays measure the host's response to infection and hence are indirect measures of infection.
- Antigen based assays are rapid, early and simple methods for the diagnosis of COVID-19.
- IgM and IgG antibodies-based assays can be used as a point of care test for assessing overall infection and immunity rates in the community.
- Large number of the population can be tested rapidly and possible community outbreak can be detected in a short time.
- The major drawbacks of serological assays are their decreased sensitivity and specificity.

Figure 5.3 depicts the appearance of SARS-CoV-2 RNA, antigen and IgM, IgG antibodies after infection.

Viral Culture
- Not recommended for diagnostic purposes.
- Can be used for research purposes such as isolation of the virus, exploring the properties of the virus and developing a vaccine.

CHALLENGES IN LABORATORY DIAGNOSIS OF COVID-19

Early diagnosis is essential for the timely management as well as isolation of confirmed cases in order to check the transmission. Sample collection, transport and kit validation are the major obstacles in the diagnosis of COVID-19. A study noted the total positivity of cases by initial RT-PCR as around 30–60%. This is dependent on the time of sample collection as PCR positivity is usually seen during the early days of symptoms. The sensitivity of the testing kits is also a matter of debate; a large number of patients may

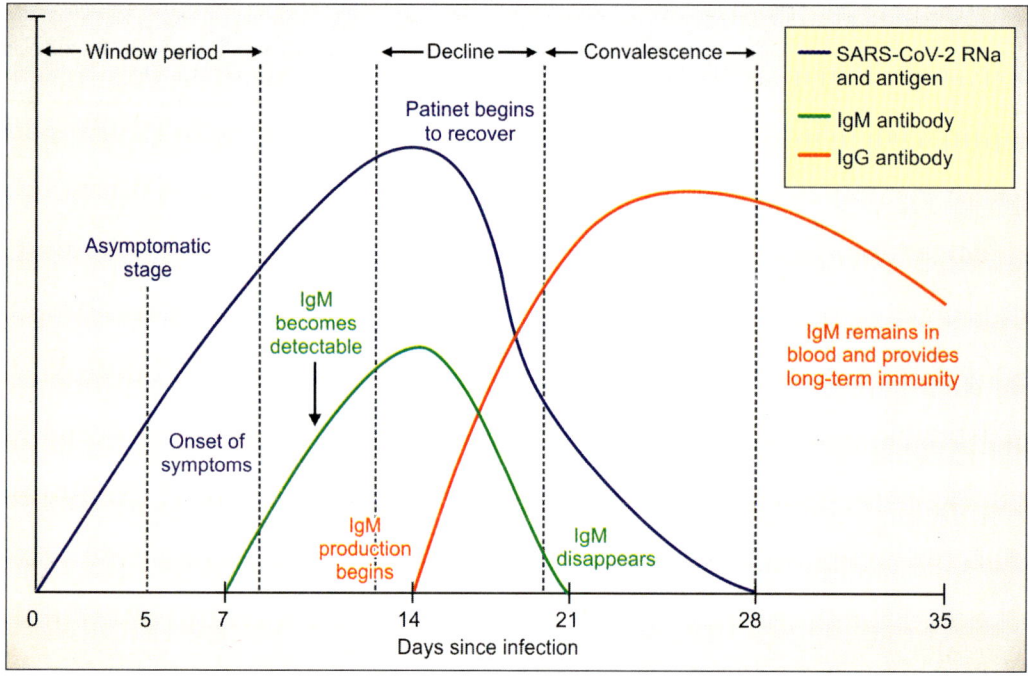

Fig. 5.3: Appearance of SARS-CoV-2 RNA, antigen and IgM, IgG antibodies after infection. (*Source:* Why do we need antibody tests for COVID-19 and how to interpret test results. In: Diazyme Laboratories. Available at: http://www.diazyme.com/covid-19-antibody-tests. Accessed Apr 13, 2020)

not be identified, which could eventually adversely affect the early diagnosis and treatment of COVID-19 patients.

In low- and middle-income countries (LMICs), the healthcare system is not strong enough. Consequently, the testing laboratories encounter difficulties in the performance of molecular testing.

FUTURE PERSPECTIVES

Considering the above challenges for diagnosis, a strong laboratory network is urgently needed. India has a wide network of laboratories for testing of viral disease; the Viral Research and Diagnostic Laboratories (VRDL) which forms the base of the pyramid with an apex center at the top. In these unprecedented times, these VRDLs are leading the real-time diagnosis of COVID-19 in India. This robust network of laboratories can be replicated in LMICs for quick sample collection to the final diagnosis of SARS-CoV-2 and other viral infections.

CHAPTER

6

Radiological Features of COVID-19 Infection

Anju Garg, Rashmi Dixit, Shruti Mittal

INTRODUCTION

Coronavirus disease-2019 (COVID-19) is an infectious viral disease caused by severe acute respiratory syndrome coronavirus 2 (SARS-CoV-2). Although this typically presents with pulmonary involvement, various non-pulmonary manifestations have increasingly been reported. The diagnosis is made on the basis of a positive RT-PCR assay.

ROLE OF IMAGING

The role of imaging lies primarily in evaluating the extent of disease (severity), disease progression, complications and for follow-up. Chest imaging is also indicated in some specific clinical situations where other associated lung pathologies like pulmonary thromboembolism, inflammatory/neoplastic diseases need to be ruled out. Chest radiographs and computed tomography (CT) are the primary imaging modalities used.

Chest Radiograph (CXR)

Plain radiograph of the chest is the first-line imaging modality for evaluation of patients known or suspected to have COVID-19. Although the sensitivity of chest radiograph is low early in the disease course, it may help in the diagnosis of moderate/severe cases of COVID-19 when the pattern of lung involvement on chest radiograph is assessed in conjunction with history, clinical presentation and laboratory parameters of the patient. Chest radiographs also help in assessing the disease severity, its progression and in post-recovery follow-up. Portable chest radiography also has a crucial role in imaging critically ill/debilitated and ICU patients. These mobile X-ray units are relatively inexpensive, easily available and can be transported to the patient's bedside or deployed in dedicated covid wards, thereby reducing the risk of exposure to infection in healthcare workers.

Indications for performing chest radiograph

In patients suspected with COVID-19 infection:
- CXRs are recommended in all patients presenting with severe acute respiratory illness (SARI).

- CXR is warranted when any two of the following are present
  - Fever
  - Shortness of breath
  - Immunocompromised status
  - Hypoxia (room air SpO_2 <94%)
  - Respiratory rate >20/minute.

In COVID-19 positive patients:
- In symptomatic RT-PCR positive patients: Periodic chest X-rays can be performed based on the clinical status of the patient; however, daily X-rays are not recommended.
- In asymptomatic RT-PCR positive patients: CXR is not recommended.

Imaging manifestations: In early/mild disease, the CXR can be normal in up to 30% patients and a normal chest radiograph does not rule out COVID-19 infection.

The chest X-ray findings are most evident after 10–12 days of symptom onset. The characteristic findings are bilateral, peripheral and lower zone predominant air space opacities seen as ground glass opacities {GGO} and/or consolidation (Figs 6.1 and 6.2). Multifocal bilateral lower zone consolidation is most easily observed while subtle findings of GGOs are less apparent and may be difficult to detect on CXR. Other findings like ill-defined nodular and linear opacities can also be seen. Based on the clinical status of the patient, serial chest radiographs can be used in assessing the disease progression and follow up (Fig. 6.3).

CXR is not a diagnostic modality for novel COVID-19 infection; the findings should be considered along with clinical parameters, history of exposure and isolation of virus in nasopharyngeal/oropharyngeal swab. Various conditions that can present with similar imaging features on CXR include other viral pneumonias, atypical bacterial

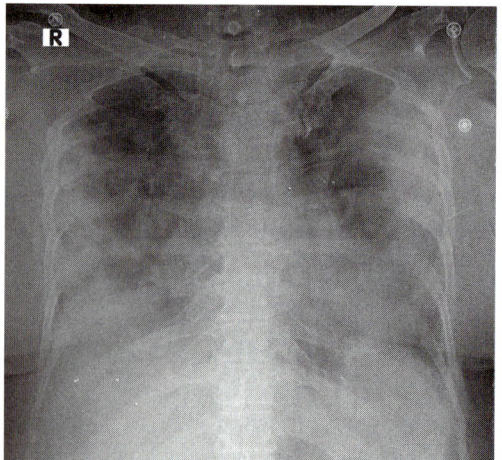 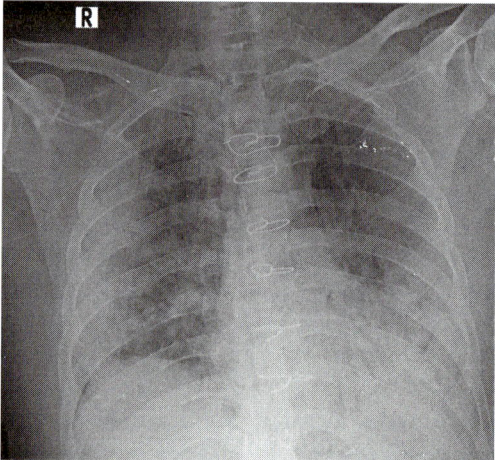

Fig. 6.1: Frontal chest radiograph in a 58-year-old COVID-19 positive patient shows multifocal peripheral areas of consolidation in bilateral lung fields with middle and lower zone and predominance. These are **typical** features of COVID 19 pneumonia.

Fig. 6.2: Frontal chest radiograph in an adult COVID-19 positive patient shows **typical pattern** of multifocal peripherally distributed airspace consolidation in bilateral mid and lower lung zones.

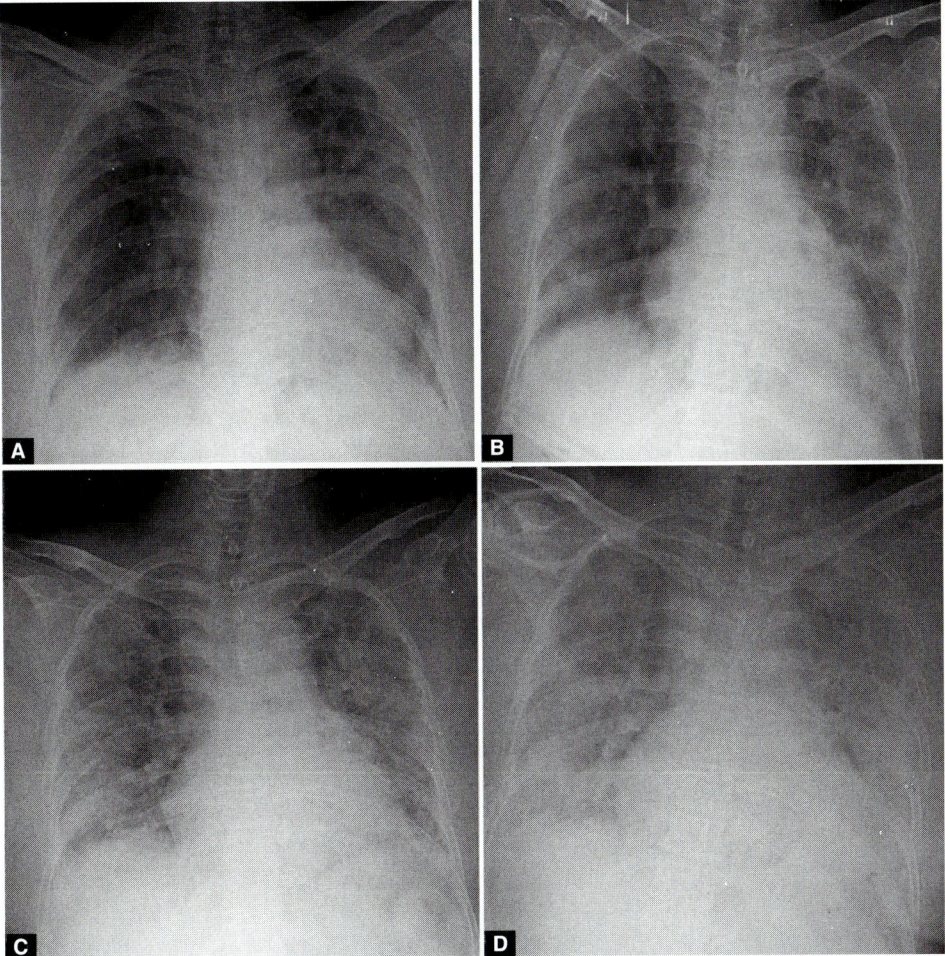

Fig. 6.3(A–D): Serial chest radiographs were performed in a 76-year-old COVID-19 patient on day 1, 4, 14 and 17 which reveal progression of the disease process.
Day 1 (A) and day 4 (B) chest radiographs show presence of ground glass haze in bilateral middle and lower zones (left > right) with peripheral predominance which progressed to multifocal peripheral areas of consolidation on day 14 (C). Chest radiograph on Day 17 (D) shows further progression of disease as confluent areas of consolidation involving bilateral lung fields.

pneumonia, non-cardiogenic pulmonary edema, intra-alveolar hemorrhage from small vessel vasculitis, and drug induced pneumonitis.

On the basis of the findings of chest radiograph, the final impression can be given as follows [reporting template proposed by British Society of Thoracic Imaging, (BSTI)]:

1. **Normal:** No findings on chest X-ray; chest radiograph can be normal in the early phase of COVID-19 pneumonia. However, normal CXR does not exclude COVID-19 infection.
2. **Classic/probable/typical COVID-19:** Bilateral multifocal lower lobe and peripheral predominant areas of GGO and/or consolidation (Fig. 6.4).

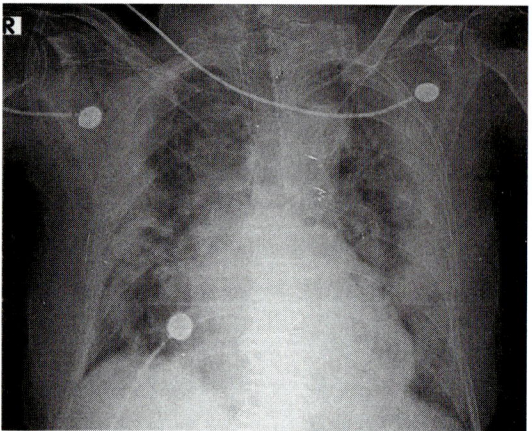

Fig. 6.4: Frontal chest radiograph in a 64-year COVID-19 positive patient shows multifocal areas of consolidation in bilateral lung fields with peripheral predominance, consistent with **typical** features of COVID-19 pneumonia.

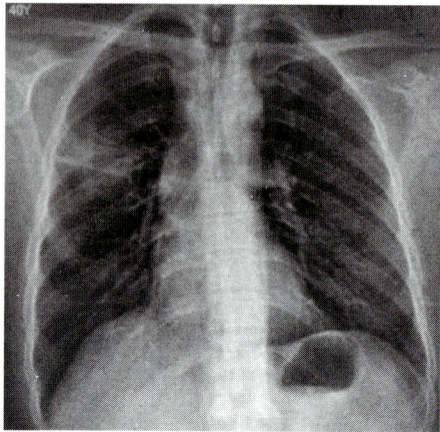

Fig. 6.5: Frontal chest radiograph in a COVID-19 suspect reveals an area of consolidation in the right middle zone. This finding is **indeterminate** for COVID-19.

3. **Indeterminate for COVID-19:** Chest X-ray are not consistent with classic COVID or non-COVID descriptors, absence of typical findings, unilateral, central and upper lobe predominant distribution (Fig. 6.5).

4. **Atypical/non-COVID-19:** Lobar pneumonia, pleural effusion, pulmonary edema, pneumothorax, solitary pulmonary nodule or diffuse tiny nodules (Figs 6.6 and 6.7).

In addition to the final impression which is based on the lung parenchymal involvement, other additional observations such as lymphadenopathy, cardiomegaly, cavities, pneumothorax, pleural effusion and atelectasis are also mentioned in the reporting template.

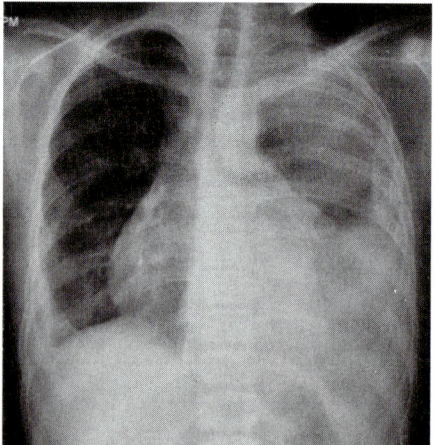

Fig. 6.6: Frontal chest radiograph in a 15-year-old COVID-19 suspect shows bilateral pleural effusion (left > right) with collapse/consolidation of underlying lung parenchyma. Findings are **atypical** for COVID-19.

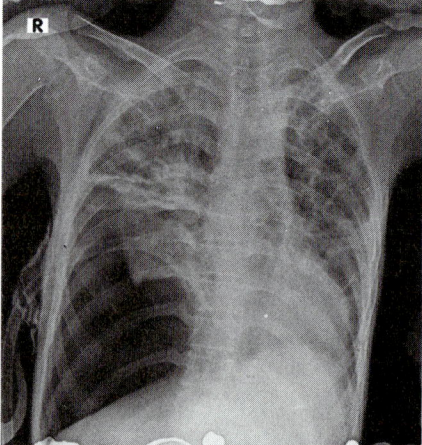

Fig. 6.7: Frontal chest radiograph in a 18-year-old COVID-19 suspect reveals right sided pneumothorax with intercostal drainage tube *in situ*; with fibrotic and fibrobronchiectatic changes in bilateral lung fields. Findings are **atypical** for COVID-19.

Based on the extent of lung involvement on the chest radiograph, scoring systems have been devised to quantify the severity/extent of disease discussed as below:

A scoring system proposed by Borghesi and Moraldi was specifically designed to be used in COVID-19 positive cases and is also known as the *Brixia score.*

This scoring system requires two step image analysis. The first step is to divide each lung into three zones on frontal chest projection (PA or AP), i.e. into 6 lung regions: Upper, middle and lower lung on each side. In the second step, a score (from 0 to 3 points) is assigned to each zone based on the detected lung abnormalities that is, 0–no lung abnormalities; (1) interstitial infiltrates; (2) interstitial and alveolar infiltrates (interstitial predominance); and (3) interstitial and alveolar infiltrates (alveolar predominance). The overall score is the sum of the points from all the zones with a range from 0 to 18 (Fig. 6.8).

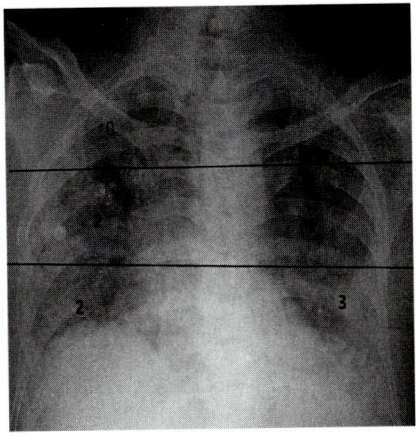

Fig. 6.8: Frontal chest radiograph of a COVID-19 positive patient reveals multifocal peripheral areas of ground glass haze and consolidation in bilateral lung fields predominantly in bilateral middle and lower zones. On assessment of lung involvement, a score of 8 points was observed in this case. (0 + 2 + 2 = 4 on the right side, 0 + 1 + 3 = 4 on the left side, both the sides were summed up, i.e. 4 + 4 and a **chest X-ray score** of 8 was assigned in this case).

The CXR score is reported to be significantly higher in patients with severe disease as compared to patients with mild disease. This semi-quantitative score helps in assessment of disease severity, progression of pulmonary involvement and is a useful parameter in predicting mortality of hospitalized patients with COVID–19 infection. In a study conducted by *Borghesi et al* in May 2020, it was observed that a chest X-ray score of more than 8 was associated with higher risk of mortality in hospitalized patients with COVID-19.

Another practical and simple chest X-ray scoring system can be used where the lung field is divided into three zones each, similar to Borghes *et al*. The score is based on the percentage of lung involvement by the disease within each zone rather than the pattern, as discussed below:

0: normal/no parenchymal involvement

1: 1–25% of area involved

2: up to 50% of area involved

3: up to 75% of area involved

4: >75% of the area involved.

The maximum score for each zone is 4 and the minimum being 0. The value of this score ranges from 0 to 24.

COMPUTED TOMOGRAPHY (CT) OF CHEST

CT has a greater sensitivity than chest radiograph in detecting COVID-19 related abnormalities and has a potential role in diagnosis under specific clinical settings, helps in predicting the prognosis and detection of complications of the disease.

Indications of Chest CT in COVID-19

CT should not be used indiscriminately as a screening modality or as a first-line test to diagnose COVID-19. Approximately 15–50% of the patients may be negative for covid pneumonia on chest CT especially in the early course of the disease. The decision for CT imaging should be made by the treating clinician, and it should be used judiciously to guide further management and to rule out suspected complications and coexisting lung pathologies. The following are the recommended indications for performing CT chest.

In patients suspected to have COVID-19: CT Chest is indicated in COVID-19 suspects having moderate to severe illness where the RT-PCR report is either negative or awaited and chest X-ray is either indeterminate or normal. CT in these patients may help in further guidance and in early and prompt management. The diagnostic accuracy of chest CT further improves when imaging findings are assessed along with various laboratory parameters, such as raised CRP, LDH, D-Dimer and serum ferritin levels.

In COVID-19 positive patients: CT is not indicated in every positive patient. It is done only in some specific clinical situations where it is expected to influence the treatment plan and further management of the patient, as mentioned below:

- Patients with sudden clinical deterioration/unresponsive to treatment.
- Patients with suspected pulmonary thromboembolism, e.g. when saturation falling disproportionately to the lung parenchymal changes may require CTPA.
- Patients with suspected concurrent other lung pathology (infective/neoplastic/inflammatory).
- Patients with high-risk of disease progression such as those with age more than 65 years, history of diabetes mellitus, history of cardiovascular disease, chronic respiratory disease, obesity, hypertension and immunocompromised status.
- Patients experiencing mild symptoms with normal/indeterminate chest X-ray and SpO_2 <93% at rest or abnormal saturation on 6 minute walk test. CT is indicated in these patients to triage them for hospitalization.
- Serial CT scans of patients are not recommended, and patients are best followed up with X-rays and clinicolaboratory parameters.

 Chest CT is not recommended for routine screening of COVID-19.

 Normal CT in the early course of the disease may lead to false impression of being covid negative and results in improper isolation of infected population. It also poses higher risk of infection both to healthcare workers as well as other patients without adding much added benefit in the patient management.

Scanning Protocol for CT Chest

Protocol: Routine HRCT/NCCT chest is acquired in volumetric mode, from thoracic inlet to the upper abdomen with patient lying in supine position with arms extended overhead in deep inspiration.

 The acquired CT images are reconstructed into soft tissue mediastinal window (20–30 kernel) and lung window (in a sharp algorithm ~80 kernel which becomes the *high-resolution CT*) and in 1.2–1.5 mm section thickness for interpretation. Iodinated contrast may be considered when indicated in certain specific circumstances, like for CT pulmonary angiography or in cases with frank hemoptysis.

Radiation dose: Currently, in standard dose/routine NCCT, the effective radiation dose is approximately 6–7 mSv. While CT imaging has been shown to be a great help in establishing the diagnosis of COVID-19, the potential for increased radiation exposure to a large number of patients cannot be ignored. Low dose CT protocols (20–40 mAs and 80–120 KVp) are now increasingly being used with reasonably good diagnostic image quality and the effective radiation dose received from low dose CT chest is approximately 1–3 mSv.

Since ground glass opacities and consolidation are primary CT presentations of COVID-19, that have been shown to be effectively picked up in LDCT, it can accurately diagnose and grade the severity of covid pneumonia and serves as an effective tool in patients requiring multiple scans. There is no significant difference between the low-dose and standard-dose CT images in diagnosing laboratory-confirmed COVID-19 pneumonia cases, with excellent agreement rate among the readers.

Imaging Findings on Chest CT in COVID-19 Patients

Terms
- Ground glass opacity (GGO): A hazy increase in lung attenuation without obscuration of the underlying bronchovascular markings. This is the most characteristic imaging finding especially when multifocal, bilateral and peripheral.
- Consolidation: There is increase in lung attenuation obscuring the underlying vessels and bronchial margins surrounded by GGO.
- Crazy paving pattern: The combination of ground glass opacity with interlobular septal thickening gives rise to this pattern.
- Vascular dilatation: There is prominence of vessels in regions of ground glass opacity (luminal dilation/engorgement or mural thickening of pulmonary vessels).
- Traction bronchiectasis.
- Subpleural bands/architectural distortion: These are thin (~1–3 mm in thickness) curvilinear opacities parallel to the pleural surface less than 1 cm deep to it.

The constellation of findings seen on CT chest can be categorized into:
1. *Typical CT findings:* A wide variety of CT findings have been reported in COVID-19 positive patients. The typical CT feature of COVID-19 pneumonia is the presence of multifocal ground glass opacities (GGOs), typically with a peripheral and subpleural distribution in bilateral lung parenchyma. The involvement of multiple lobes, particularly the lower lobes is seen in the majority of patients. These areas of GGO may be superimposed with areas of focal consolidation and associated with intralobular reticulations, resulting in a crazy paving pattern (Figs 6.9 and 6.10). Consolidation predominant pattern is seen in late and complicated stages (Figs 6.10 to 6.12). Linear consolidations and other signs suggesting organizing pneumonia such as the "reverse halo" sign (i.e. areas of ground-glass opacity surrounded by peripheral consolidation) are very frequently observed, mostly in patients in later stages of disease. "Melted sugar" sign refers to gradual decrease in density of consolidation and turning into GGO, which is seen in late and remission phases.
2. *Fairly typical CT findings:* Some findings on chest CT have been described as fairly typical for COVID-19. These include; single ground glass opacity in lower lobes in the early stage of disease, pure consolidation without GGO and white lung

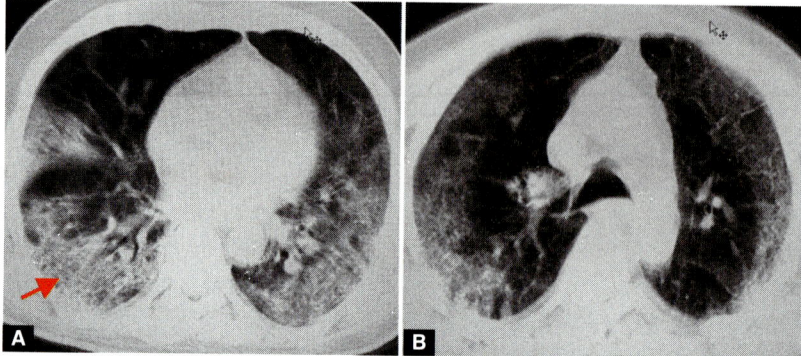

Fig. 6.9A and B: Axial non-contrast CT chest images in lung window of a 74-year-old COVID-19 suspect show **typical appearance** with confluent areas of consolidation, ground glass opacities along with **crazy paving pattern** (arrow) in bilateral peripheral lung parenchyma with basal predominance. (**CO-RADS-5**–very high suspicion for covid-19 infection).

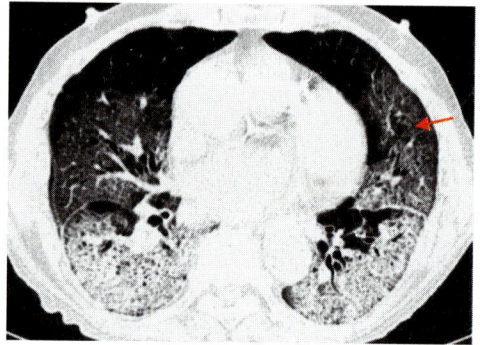

Fig. 6.10: In a similar case of a 60-year-old COVID-19 positive patient, axial non-contrast CT chest image in lung window reveals confluent ground glass opacities with superimposed reticular pattern giving **crazy paving** appearance (arrow) and areas of consolidation in bilateral lung parenchyma with peripheral predominance.

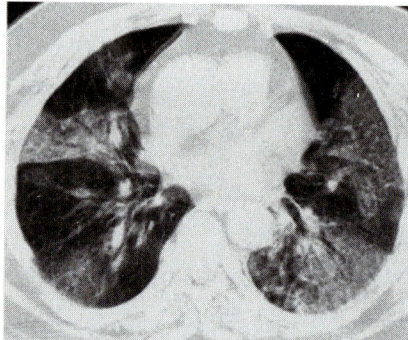

Fig. 6.11: Axial non-contrast CT chest image in lung window of a 70-year-old COVID-19 suspect shows multiple sharply marginated areas of ground glass opacity in bilateral lung parenchyma with predominant peripheral distribution. This is a classical appearance of COVID-19. (**CO-RADS 5**– very high suspicion for COVID-19).

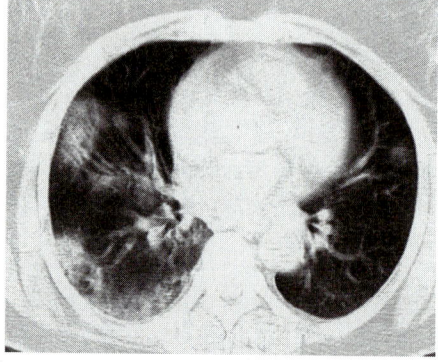

Fig. 6.12: Axial non-contrast CT chest image in a 55-year-old COVID-19 positive patient shows multifocal peripheral GGO with rounded appearance in bilateral lung parenchyma. Superimposed consolidation also noted in some of the ground glass opacities on the right side.

parenchyma in late and complicated stages. Other findings like focal pleural thickening, vascular enlargement, air bronchogram, bronchial wall thickening, and parenchymal fibrotic bands (late/remission phase) are also seen in some cases of COVID-19 (Fig. 6.13).

3. *Atypical CT findings:* These findings are inconsistent with COVID-19 and raise the suspicion for other pathologies (Fig. 6.14). These findings include; isolated lobar/segmental consolidation, cavitation, small discrete pulmonary nodules (centrilobular/tree-in-bud/peribronchovascular distribution), pleural effusion, mediastinal lymphadenopathy, "Halo" sign (nodule/consolidation with surrounding ground glass opacity), bronchiectasis, mucoid impaction in airways, pulmonary emphysema, pulmonary fibrosis, pneumothorax, and pericardial effusion.

The imaging findings on CT evolve over the course of disease. With increase in time gap between the onset of symptoms and initial chest CT evaluation, certain imaging findings like consolidation, bilateral and peripheral lung disease, greater total lung involvement, linear fibrotic opacities, the crazy-paving pattern and reverse halo sign are observed with increasing frequency.

Changes in CT findings associated with COVID-19 from the time of initial diagnosis till the patient's recovery are summarized as below:

1. **Early disease (0–4 days):** CT is either normal or the only abnormality is ground glass opacity which is observed in up to 40% of cases. Most commonly seen in peripheral, posterior and bilateral distribution.

2. **Progressive disease (5–8 days):** There is increase in size and number of ground glass opacities with accompanying interlobular septal thickening giving rise to crazy paving appearance. Presence of consolidation can be observed in almost 55% of cases. The involvement is seen in multiple lobes with lower lobe and peripheral predominance.

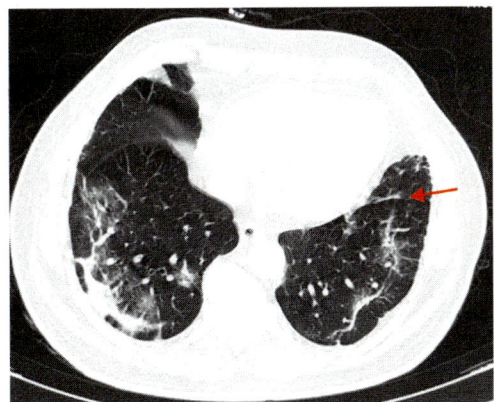

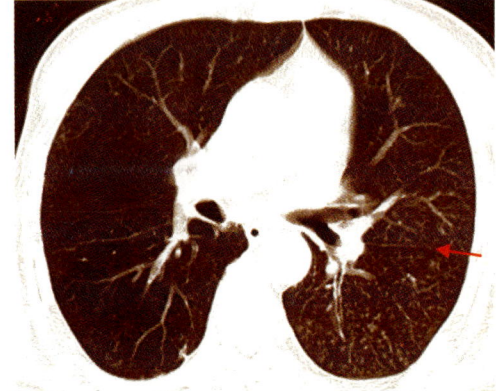

Fig. 6.13: Axial non-contrast CT chest image in lung window of a COVID-19 positive patient in the resolving phase shows multiple subpleural fibrotic opacities and linear stripes (arrow) in bilateral basal lung parenchyma and associated persistent GGOs.

Fig. 6.14: Axial non-contrast CT chest image in lung window of a 55-year-old patient with history of fever and cough shows multiple tiny centrilobular nodules in tree in bud pattern (arrow) of arrangement in the superior segment of the left lower lobe. These findings are **atypical** for COVID-19 related pneumonia and suggest another diagnosis. (**CO-RADS 2**–low suspicion for COVID-19).

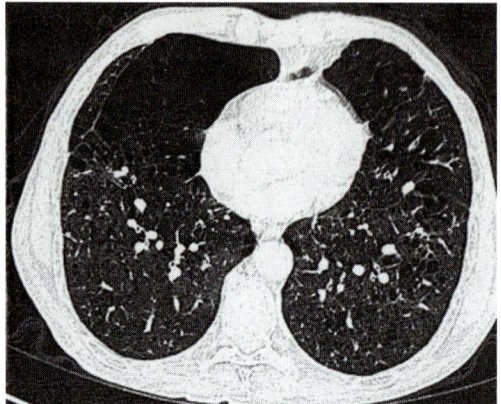

Fig. 6.15: Axial non-contrast CT chest image in lung window of a 65-year-old patient with history of smoking and breathlessness reveals paraseptal and centriacinar emphysematous changes with few fibrotic opacities in bilateral lung parenchyma (**CO-RADS 1**–very low suspicion for COVID-19/non infectious).

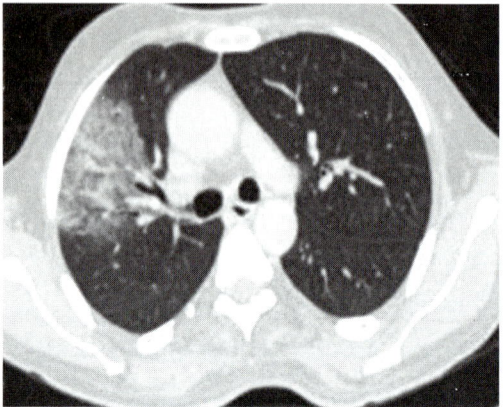

Fig. 6.16: Axial non-contrast CT chest image in lung window of a 21-year HIV positive patient old patient with complaints of fever and cough with sputum shows an area of consolidation in anterior segment of right upper lobe with air bronchograms within. This patient was later confirmed to have Klebsiella pneumonia. (**CO-RADS 2**–low suspicion for COVID-19).

3. **Peak disease (9–13 days):** Multifocal areas of consolidation, bronchial wall thickening, vascular dilatation develop in addition to the above described findings. Reverse halo sign, i.e. central area of ground glass opacity surrounded by consolidation is observed during this phase of the disease.
4. **Resolving disease (>14 days):** Fibrotic bands, subpleural lines (Fig. 6.13) and stripes begin to appear as the lung heals with reduction or disappearance of ground glass opacities and consolidation.
   - Consolidation (vs GGO) on CT is an indicator for poor prognosis.
   - Normal CT does not rule out COVID-19 infection, so CT of the chest should not be used as a screening tool.

THE COVID-19 REPORTING AND DATA SYSTEM (CO-RADS)

The CO-RADS assessment scheme was developed by the Dutch Radiological Society in patients with moderate to severe symptoms of COVID-19. It provides a level of suspicion for pulmonary involvement in patients suspected of having COVID-19 disease based on the features observed at non-contrast chest CT. It is not a scoring system and is not related to the severity/extent of the disease. CO-RADS makes provision for standardized reporting, helps in comparison of data across different institutions and thereby improves communication with referring physicians. There are 7 categories of CO-RADS ranging from 0 to 6 (Table 6.1). Category 1 to 6 follow an increasing risk for COVID-19, that is from very low risk (CO-RADS-1) to proven infection by RT-PCR positive assay (CO-RADS-6).

CO-RADS provides a standardized assessment for reporting non-contrast chest CT scans of patients with suspected COVID-19. It has excellent inter-observer agreement and good performance in discriminating cases with low or high risk for the disease.

TABLE 6.1: CO-RADS categories with the corresponding level of suspicion for pulmonary involvement in COVID-19

	Level of suspicion for pulmonary involvement of COVID-19	Summary
CO-RADS 0	Not interpretable	Scan technically insufficient for assigning a score.
CO-RADS 1	Very low	Normal or non-infectious (emphysema, perifissural nodules, lung tumors or fibrosis; Fig. 6.15).
CO-RADS 2	Low	Typical for other infections but not COVID-19 (such as bronchitis, bronchopneumonia, or lung abscess). Radiological features like lobar/segmental consolidation, tree in bud, centrilobular nodular pattern and cavities suggest disease other than COVID-19 (Fig. 6.16).
CO-RADS 3	Equivocal/unsure	Features compatible with COVID-19, that can also be found in other viral pneumonia or non-infectious diseases. Findings in this category are perihilar GGOs, GGOs with interstitial thickening with or without pleural effusion and patterns of organising pneumonia.
CO-RADS 4	High	Typical for COVID-19 but have some overlap with other viral pneumonias. Findings are similar to CO-RADS 5 but with an atypical distribution, lack of contact with the visceral pleura, strictly unilateral, predominantly peribronchovascular distribution or findings are superimposed on severe/ diffuse pre-existing pulmonary changes.
CO-RADS 5	High suspicion	Findings are typical for COVID-19, can be divided into 2 groups, i.e. mandatory features and confirmatory patterns. *Mandatory features:* • Ground-glass opacities, with or without consolidation, near visceral pleural surfaces • Multifocal bilateral distribution. *Confirmatory patterns:* • Ground-glass areas with sharp/unsharp demarcation outlining multiple adjacent secondary pulmonary lobules • Intralobular interstitial thickening with ground-glass opacities giving a "crazy paving" pattern (Fig. 6.9 to 6.11) • The pattern can evolve to resemble organizing pneumonia, giving the "reverse halo" sign with presence of curvilinear subpleural bands.
CO-RADS 6	Proven	RT-PCR positive for SARS-CoV-2

CT Severity Score

In order to standardize and quantify the radiological examinations, different algorithms for evaluating the severity of lung involvement have been proposed. The two popularly used scoring systems are discussed below:

The most commonly used method for assessing the CT severity score was presented by Li *et al.* with values ranging from 0–25 (score of 0 corresponds to no parenchymal involvement whereas, score of 25 corresponds to involvement of almost the entire lung parenchyma). This score was intended to find another objective method to identify significant radiological differences between severe and milder cases of COVID-19. The cut-off value for identifying severe cases of COVID-19 of CT score was 7, with the sensitivity and specificity of 80.0% and 82.8%, respectively.

The severity score was calculated based on lung involvement percentage (Figs 6.17 and 6.18) for each patient by scoring the percentage of each lobe involvement individually and given a score from 1 to 5 where,

Score 1: <5% involvement

Score 2: 5–25% involvement

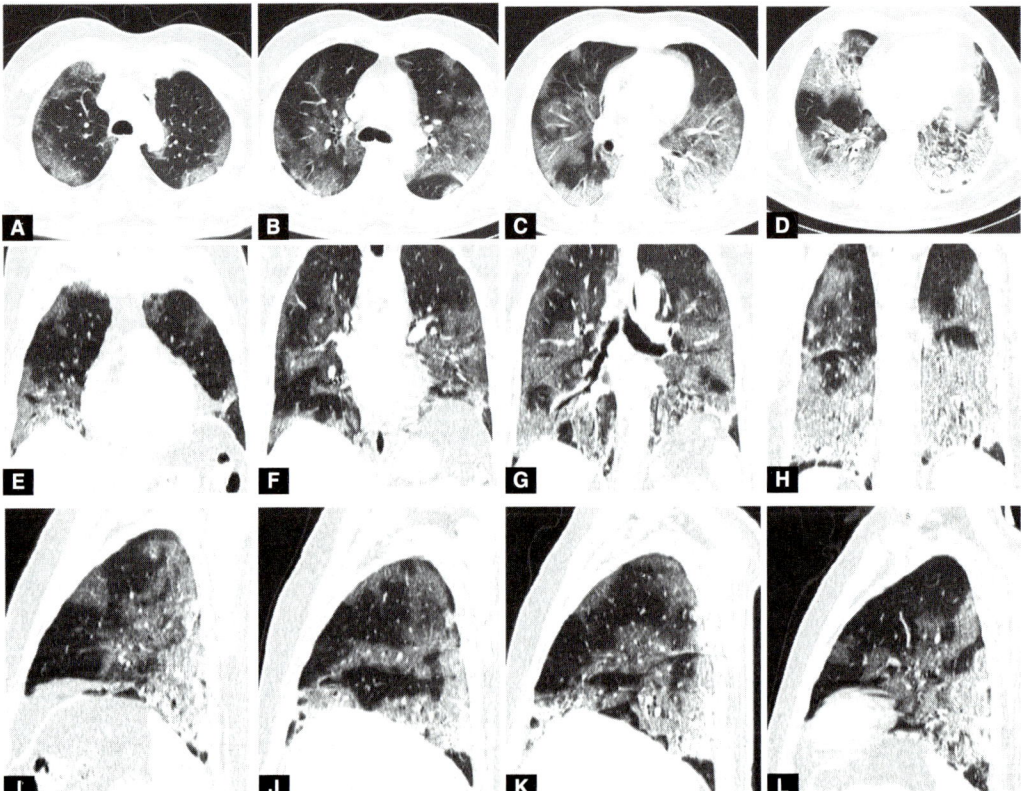

Fig. 6.17A to L: Axial (A to D), sagittal (E to H) and coronal (I to L) CT chest images in lung window of a COVID-19 positive patient, reveal multifocal peripheral ground glass opacities with areas of consolidation and interlobular septal thickening in bilateral lung parenchyma predominantly in bilateral lower lobes. The extent of lung involvement in each lobe was assessed subjectively and a CT score of 20/25 was assigned [Right upper lobe—3 (25–50%), Right middle lobe—4 (50–75%), Right lower lobe—5 (>75%), Left upper lobe—3 (25–50%) and Left lower lobe—5 (>75%)].

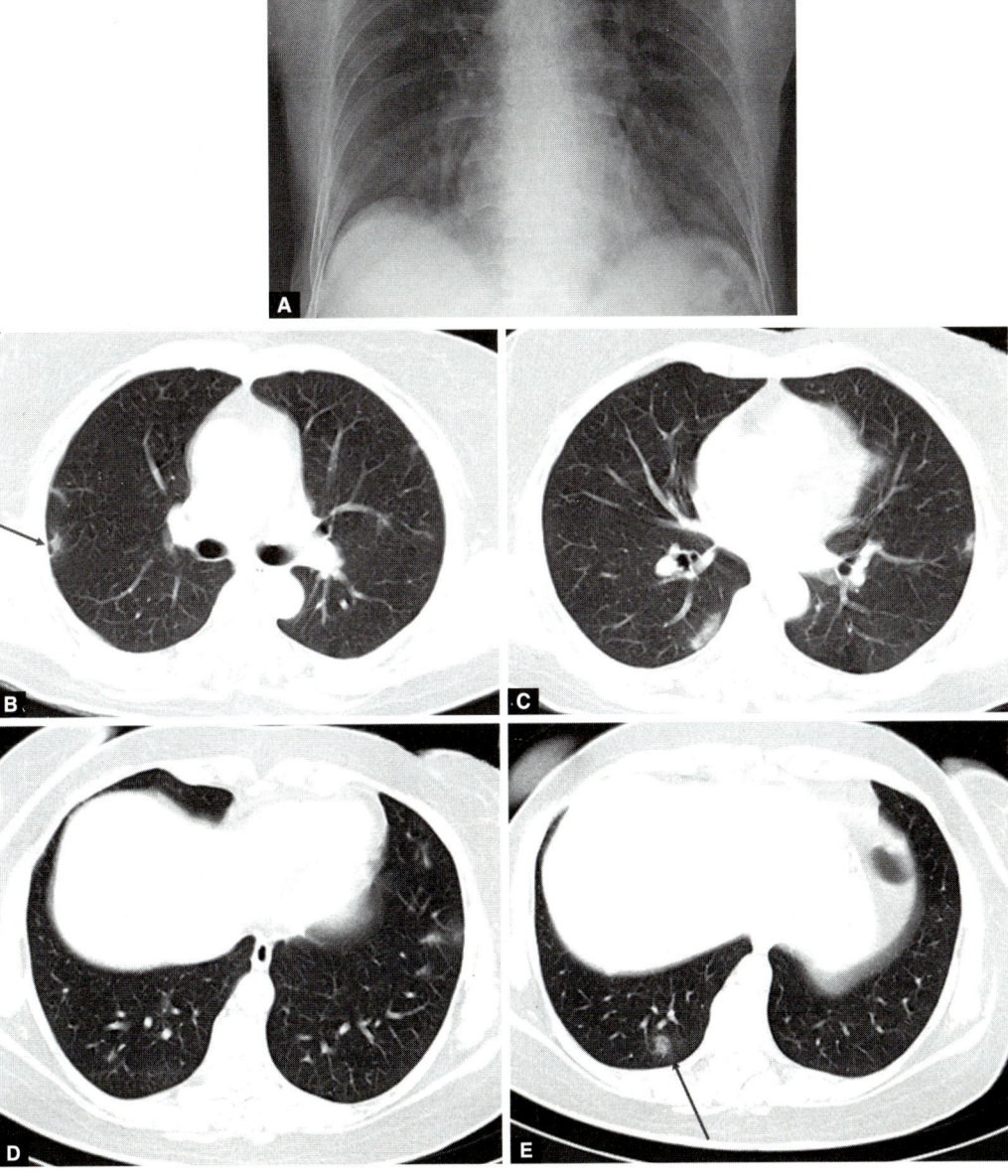

Fig. 6.18A to E: Frontal chest radiograph (A) in a 35-year-old COVID-19 positive patient appears unremarkable. Axial non-contrast CT chest images in lung window (B–E) of the same patient reveal few multifocal ground glass opacities (arrows) in bilateral upper and lower lobes (CT severity score—4/25).

Score 3: 26–50% involvement

Score 4: 51–75% involvement

Score 5: >75% involvement

Then, the final score is the sum of individual lobar scores and ranges from 0 to 25 points; the total lung involvement is then obtained by multiplying the total score by 4. CT score is positively correlated with age, inflammatory biomarkers, severity of clinical categories, and disease phases (Table 6.2). CT score ≥18 has shown to be highly predictive of patient mortality in short term follow-up.

Another method for calculating CT severity score was proposed by Yang *et al.* and was created to help in assessment of COVID-19 burden on the initial scan and to provide an objective approach for identifying patients in need of hospital admission. The score (CT-SS) is an adaptation of a previously used method during the SARS epidemic.

The 18 bronchopulmonary segments of both lungs were divided into 20 regions according to the anatomical structure, in which the posterior apical segment of the left upper lobe was subdivided into apical and posterior segments, whereas the anteromedial basal segment of the left lower lobe was subdivided into anterior and basal segments.

The lung involvement in all of these 20 lung regions were subjectively evaluated on chest CT images using scores of 0, 1, and 2 if parenchymal opacification involved 0%, less than 50%, or equal to or more than 50% of each region, respectively. The CT-SS is defined as the sum of the individual scores in the 20 lung segment regions, ranging from 0 to 40 points.

This is a semiquantitative method for assessing severity of COVID-19 in the initial chest CT images. A CT-SS score less than 19.5 could rule out severe or critical forms of disease with a high negative predictive value of 96.3%.

Imaging in the Post COVID-19 Patient

In the post recovery phase of COVID-19, it is not uncommon to have patients presenting with long-term respiratory consequences like breathlessness and/or hypoxia and deranged pulmonary function test (PFT) results. Chest CT is needed in these patients to rule out fibrotic lung disease, which is a known sequelae of COVID-19 infection.

A study was conducted by *Liu et al* in May 2020 and it was observed that pulmonary lesions were completely absorbed in 53.0% of patients during the 3rd week after discharge. They also observed that more than 40% of patients demonstrated residual abnormalities, including GGOs and fibrous stripe as the main CT manifestations at the 3-week radiological follow-up, for whom further radiological follow-up was continued. Another study was conducted by *Han et al*, which demonstrated that approximately 35% of patients who recovered from severe COVID-19 illness revealed fibrotic opacities in lung parenchyma on long term follow up of 6 months duration. It

TABLE 6.2: CT score based on extent of lung involvement and severity of the disease	
CT score	*Severity*
7 or less	Mild
8–17	Moderate
18 or more	Severe

was also observed that patients with age more than 50 years, greater duration of hospital stay (>17 days), history of mechanical ventilation, acute respiratory distress syndrome and CT severity score of more than 18 at initial presentation were independent predictors of developing fibrotic changes in the lung after 6 months follow-up.

CT imaging features such as bronchovascular bundle distortion, fibrotic stripes, traction bronchiectasis, architectural distortion, and interlobular septal thickening are suggestive of pulmonary fibrosis (Fig. 6.19). Fibrosis has been more commonly seen in patients with severe symptoms and a higher level of inflammatory markers, including interleukin-6 and C-reactive protein. Interstitial thickening, coarse reticular pattern, irregular interfaces, and parenchymal bands seen at CT during the acute phase of the disease may be indicators of impending pulmonary fibrosis and need to be evaluated carefully. This group of patients need multidisciplinary care with assessment of radiographic and physiologic pulmonary abnormalities which may help in early medical treatment strategies such as antifibrotic drugs, thus reducing disease morbidity and mortality rates.

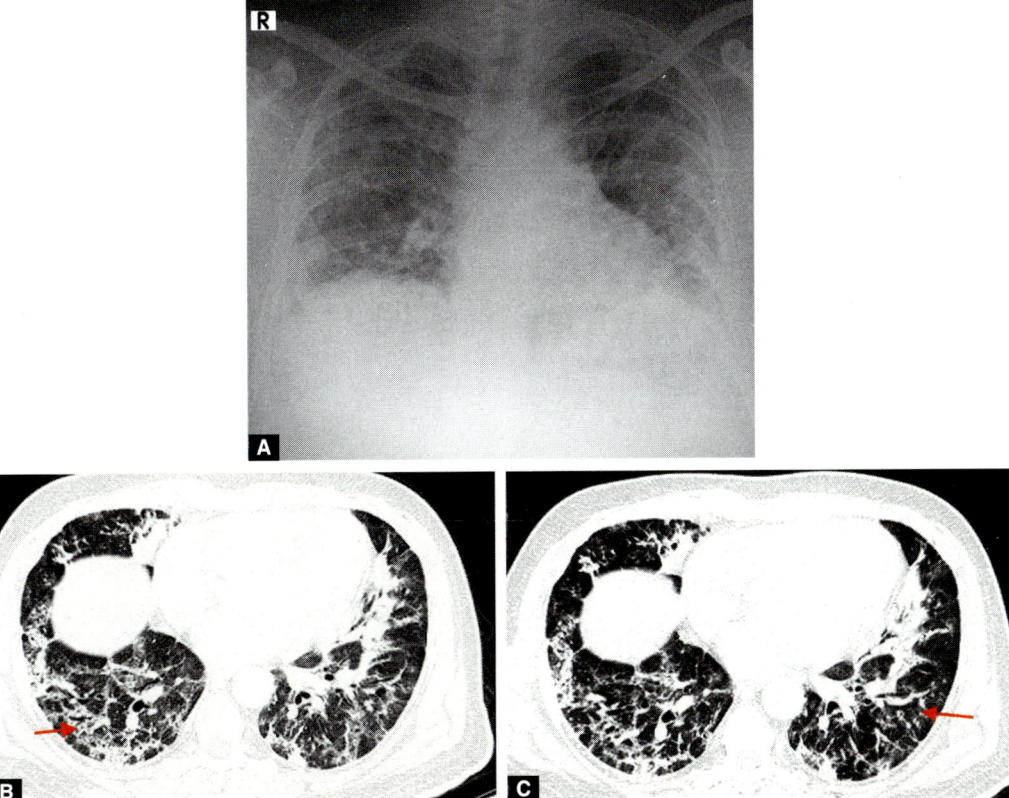

Fig. 6.19A to C: Frontal chest radiograph (A) performed after 3 weeks in a COVID-19 recovered patient, reveals prominent interstitial markings with fibrotic opacities predominantly in bilateral middle and lower zones (arrow). Axial non-contrast CT images in lung window (B, C) of the same patient reveal fibrotic parenchymal bands predominantly in bilateral lower lobes with associated mild cylindrical tractional bronchiectasis (long arrow), and interlobular septal thickening (short arrow).

Extrapulmonary Manifestations and Complications of COVID-19

Vascular Manifestations

Prothrombotic complications have been recognized as a feature of COVID-19. Solid organ infarcts may be visualized at abdominal imaging in patients with COVID-19, affecting the kidney, spleen, and liver. At Doppler ultrasound, decreased vascularity within a solid organ is indicative of an infarct, and in these cases, it is essential to assess the primary vasculature of the affected organ for the presence of a thrombus. Vascular thrombosis may be seen as a filling defect within one or more of the supplying vessels at CT and US. Contrast-enhanced CT images may show a hypoattenuating wedge-shaped area in the solid organ parenchyma, corresponding to the infarct.

Pulmonary Vascular Manifestations

There is an increased incidence of acute pulmonary thromboembolism and other thrombotic events amongst patients with COVID-19 infection. "Dilated vessel" sign is commonly observed on non-contrast CT chest which may be attributed to increased pulmonary blood flow, small pulmonary embolism or *in situ* pulmonary venous thrombosis. It has been demonstrated in various studies that clots and thrombotic lesions disproportionately involve the distal pulmonary vasculature with lower than expected rate of proximal pulmonary artery involvement and concurrent deep vein thrombosis. Imaging is also helpful in diagnosing deep vein thrombosis and pulmonary thromboembolism. Acute pulmonary embolism is seen as a filling defect within the pulmonary vasculature and the embolus typically makes an acute angle with the vessel wall. In the axial plane, the central filling defect from the thrombus is surrounded by a thin rim of contrast which is known as the "polo mint" sign.

Neurological Manifestations

Neurological illness is a relatively common manifestation of COVID-19 seen in overall 5% of cases. However, in the critically ill patients and in ICU settings, approximately 20% of patients will have some type of neurological impairment. The most common clinical symptoms include anosmia, headache, confusion, and encephalopathy.

Approximately half of the patients who undergo neuroimaging in the setting of COVID-19 reveal various pattern of abnormal findings, as mentioned below:
- Cerebral micro-hemorrhages
- Acute spontaneous intracranial hemorrhage (ICH)
- Acute to subacute infarcts
- Encephalitis or encephalopathy
- Meningitis.

Since the majority of neuro-imaging findings in these patients are nonspecific, it remains unclear whether they are related to the underlying infection or to the multiple confounding comorbidities, including prolonged hypoxia and deranged coagulation parameters.

Cardiac Manifestations

COVID-19 patients may present with acute myocardial injury, myocarditis, coronary artery aneurysms, shock and arrhythmias. Imaging in these conditions may manifest as cardiomegaly, pericardial effusion and features of pulmonary edema. Contrast enhanced MRI in myocarditis reveals altered T1/T2 signals, lower left ventricular ejection fraction, high left ventricular volumes with early and late gadolinium enhancement in the subepicardial region.

Gastrointestinal Manifestations

A significant number of patients present with gastrointestinal complaints, mostly in the form of diarrhea. Nausea, vomiting and abdominal pain are the other symptoms. On plain abdominal radiographs, presence of generalized bowel distension with air-fluid levels may be seen, producing an ileus pattern. Contrast-enhanced CT can show thickening and edema with hyper enhancement of bowel wall predominantly involving the colorectal and small bowel loops. Fluid filled distended intestinal loops with surrounding fat stranding are also observed.

Hepatobiliary Manifestation

Elevated liver enzymes signifying liver injury can be seen in COVID-19 patients. Hepatic steatosis in the form of increased liver parenchymal echogenicity on ultrasound and hypodense liver parenchyma on CT may be seen in such cases. Periportal edema and heterogeneity of liver parenchyma on cross sectional imaging should raise a concern for hepatitis.

Biliary stasis and cholestasis are known complications of COVID-19 which can manifest as intrahepatic bile duct dilatation, dilatation of gallbladder with presence of sludge and stones within (Fig. 6.20).

Pancreatic injury has also been reported in cases of COVID-19 which may occur due to direct cytopathic effects or indirect involvement of pancreas by systemic inflammatory response. On CT scan, pancreas may appear bulky, heterogeneous with peripancreatic fat stranding and peripancreatic fluid collections.

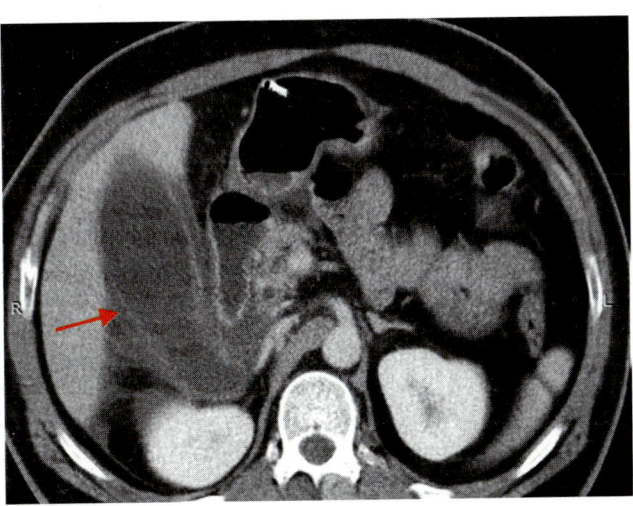

Fig. 6.20: Axial contrast enhanced CT scan image of the upper abdomen in a COVID-19 positive patient with abdominal pain reveals overdistended gallbladder with edematous walls, pericholecystic fluid and adjacent fat stranding (arrow) suggestive of acute cholecystitis.

Renal Manifestations

Acute renal failure with elevated plasma creatinine levels may be seen in critically ill COVID-19 patients. Ultrasound features of acute renal failure (such as increased parenchymal echogenicity and loss of corticomedullary differentiation) can be seen in these cases. Contrast imaging should be performed with caution in these patients. In cases of renal infarction, hypoperfusion of the renal parenchyma and wedge-shaped areas of decreased perfusion and/or enhancement may be visualized at US and contrast-enhanced CT (Fig. 6.21).

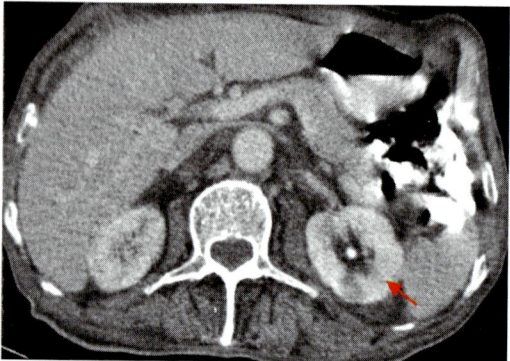

Fig. 6.21: Axial contrast enhanced CT section through lumbar region in a 77-year-old COVID-19 positive male patient reveals a wedge shaped hypodense area involving the posterior aspect of the mid pole of left kidney suggestive of renal infarct (arrow).

COVID-19 ASSOCIATED MUCORMYCOSIS (CAM)

COVID-19 is associated with significant risk of secondary fungal and bacterial infections due to immune dysregulation. With the widespread use of steroids, antibiotics and monoclonal antibodies in the treatment of COVID-19, there is development or exacerbation of pre-existing fungal disease especially in patients having diabetes mellitus or immunocompromised status. Invasive pulmonary aspergillosis is a well recognized complication of COVID-19. Currently, there is a surge in cases of COVID-19 associated with mucormycosis presenting most commonly with rhino-orbito-cerebral involvement followed by pulmonary involvement. Imaging in mucormycosis helps in early diagnosis, evaluation of the extent of disease and plays a crucial role in initiating prompt treatment.

Rhino-orbitocerebral mucormycosis (ROCM) is the most common site for CAM. Imaging features are nonspecific. CT scan of paranasal sinuses in cases of ROCM may demonstrate presence of nodular mucosal thickening with absence of fluid levels, periantral fat stranding and effacement, presence of hyperdense contents with erosions of the bony orbital walls, invasion of recti muscles and nasal septal perforation in the later course of the disease. Cross sectional imaging helps in evaluating intracranial and intraorbital extension of disease, skull base invasion, perineural spread and vascular involvement. The paranasal sinuses reveal variable appearance depending on the presence of fungal elements in sinus contents with heterogeneous post contrast enhancement (Fig. 6.22). Nasal turbinates may be bulky and swollen and the devitalized mucosa appears as patchy areas of non-enhancing tissue referred to as the 'black turbinate sign'.

Orbital involvement can result in cellulitis, orbital abscess and subperiosteal abscess. Extraocular muscle may be involved which appear bulky and show adjacent fat stranding on cross sectional imaging (Figs 6.22 and 6.23). Heterogeneously enhancing soft tissue can be observed in the preorbital region, in the extra/intraconal compartment of the orbit and along the orbital apex which can extend into the cavernous sinus leading to its thrombosis.

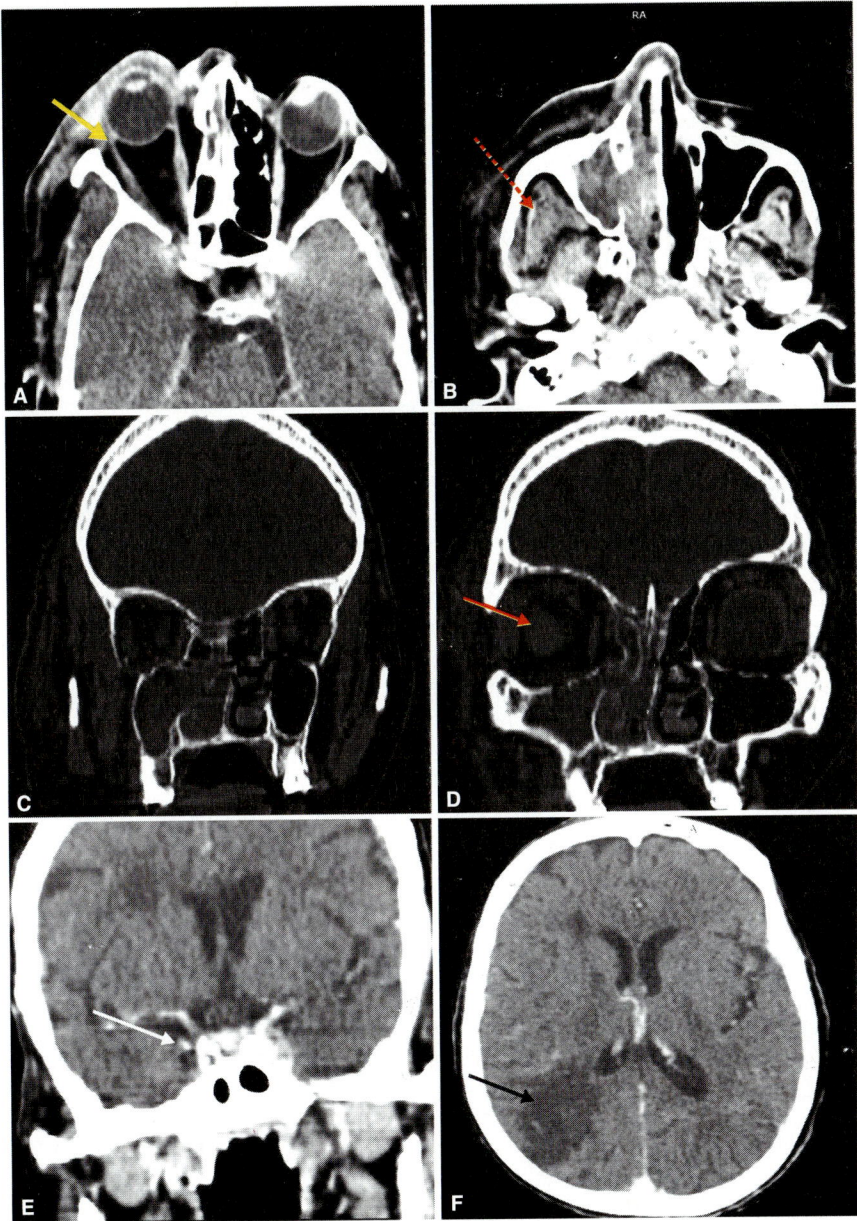

Fig. 6.22A to F: Axial contrast enhanced CT soft tissue (A, B) and coronal bone window images (C,D) in a 64-year-old COVID-19 patient with clinically suspected invasive fungal sinusitis reveal soft tissue contents in the right maxillary sinus (dotted arrow) associated with rarefaction of the medial wall of right maxillary sinus, right inferior and middle turbinates (red arrow) with extension into the right nasal cavity and ethmoidal air cells. Enhancing soft tissue thickening is also noted involving the right preseptal and preorbital region (yellow arrow) with associated fat stranding extending into the right infratemporal region. Coronal soft tissue image of the same patient (E) shows no postcontrast enhancement of the right cavernous sinus (white arrow) suggestive of cavernous sinus thrombosis. Axial CT head image (F) reveals ill-defined hypoattenuating areas in right parieto-occipital (black arrow) and centrum semiovale with loss of gray white matter interface suggestive of infarcts. Patient was diagnosed as invasive fungal sinusitis with cavernous sinus thrombosis and brain infarct.

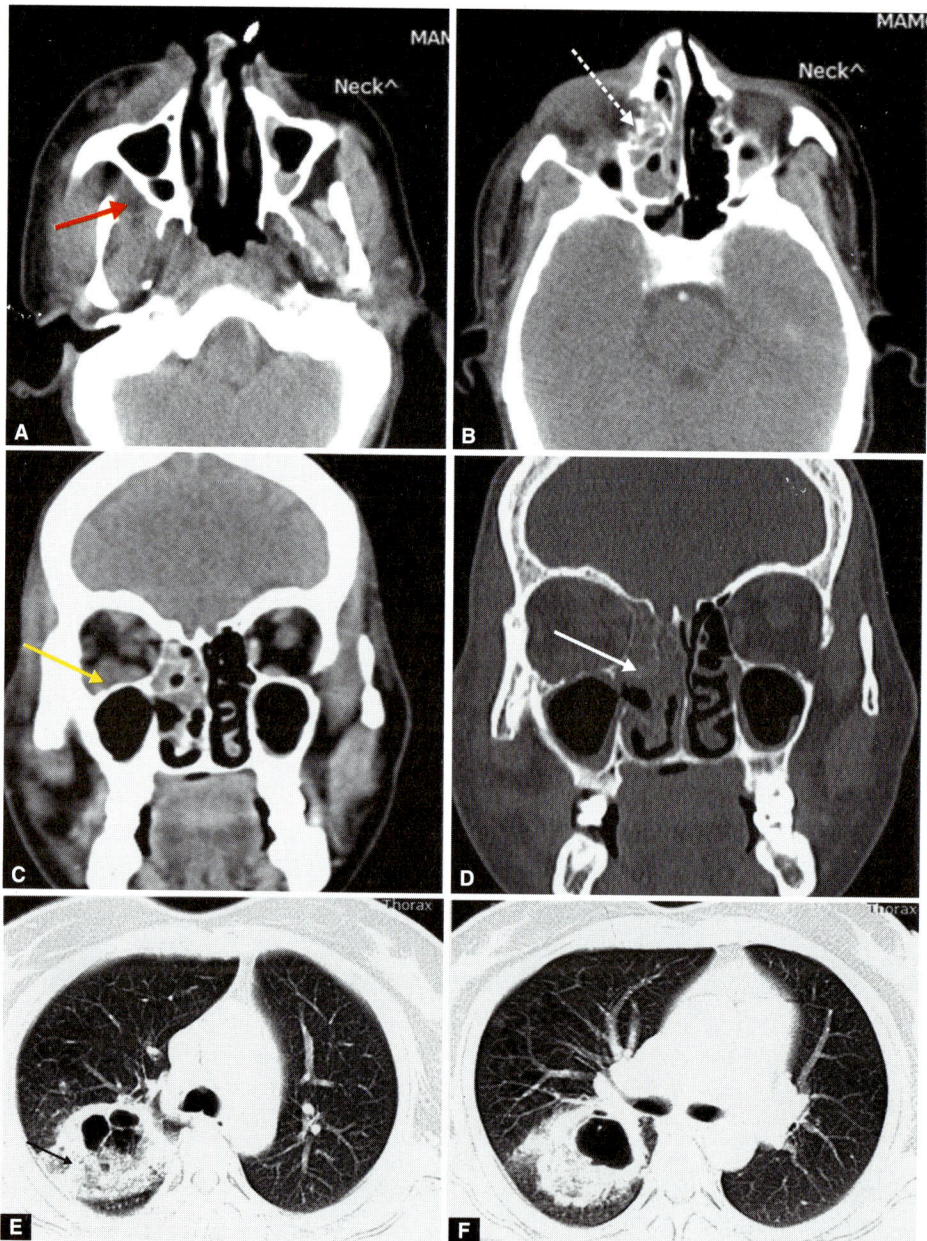

Fig. 6.23A to F: Contrast enhanced axial (A,B) and coronal soft tissue (C) and bone window (D) images of paranasal sinuses in A 37-year-old type 2 diabetic patient with history of cough, sudden onset right sided proptosis and facial swelling, reveal soft tissue thickening along the right premaxillary region with effacement of fat in the retroantral region (red arrows); mucosal thickening in the right ethmoidal air cells (dotted arrow) causing rarefaction of the ethmoidal trabeculae (white arrow) with bulky and heterogeneous right extraocular muscles (yellow arrow). Axial NCCT images in lung window (E,F) of the same patient reveal a thick walled cavity in right upper lobe with few septations and ground glass opacities in the center with surrounding area of consolidation, nodules and ground glass haze giving rise to "reverse halo" appearance (arrow). The patient underwent biopsy during nasal endoscopy and was diagnosed as rhino-orbital mucormycosis with pulmonary involvement.

Intracranial extension with involvement of the brain parenchyma can lead to formation of abscesses predominantly involving the frontal and temporal lobes.

Vascular invasion and thrombosis is a common complication of rhino-orbitocerebral mucormycosis. Heterogeneous soft tissue at the orbit apex extending into the cavernous sinus with lack of enhancement on post contrast scans suggest cavernous sinus thrombosis. Involvement of the internal carotid artery can result in ischemia and infarction (Fig. 6.22).

Imaging in pulmonary mucormycosis: On CT chest, in the early phase of the disease perivascular GGOs may be observed which progress to consolidation, nodules or masses. Mucormycosis has a high tendency for vascular invasion resulting in necrosis and relative paucity of air bronchograms in consolidation. Rarely, the lesions can invade the central vasculature leading to frank hemoptysis. There are certain imaging pointers which favor the diagnosis of pulmonary mucormycosis over invasive pulmonary aspergillosis such as presence of multiple lesions (>10), pleural effusions, large ground glass halo and 'reverse halo sign' (Fig. 6.23). The "reverse halo" sign on CT is one of the most important signs in pulmonary mucormycosis and is more commonly observed in patients with neutropenia. Organizing pneumonia, pulmonary infarct and lung cancer are important differential diagnosis for this appearance. The disease can spread to involve the chest wall, mediastinum, pleura and the diaphragm.

BIBLIOGRAPHY

1. Agrawal R, Yeldandi A, Savas H, Parekh N, Lombardi P, Hart E. Pulmonary Mucormycosis: Risk Factors, Radiologic Findings, and Pathologic Correlation. RadioGraphics. 2020;40(3):656–66.
2. Ali R, Ghonimy M. Post-COVID-19 pneumonia lung fibrosis: a worrisome sequelae in surviving patients. Egyptian Journal of Radiology and Nuclear Medicine. 2021;52(1).
3. Behzad S, Aghaghazvini L, Radmard AR, Gholamrezanezhad A. Extrapulmonary manifestations of COVID-19: Radiologic and clinical overview./*Clin Imaging.* 2020;66:35–41.
4. Bhalla AS, Jana M, Naranje P, Manchanda S. Role of Chest Radiographs during COVID-19 Pandemic. Ann Natl Acad Med Sci. 2020;56(03):138–44.
5. Bhalla AS, Raj V, Mahajan A, et al. Imaging Recommendation by Indian Radiological and Imaging Association (IRIA) and Indian College of Radiology and Imaging (ICRI) for COVID-19.
6. Borghesi A, Maroldi R. COVID-19 outbreak in Italy: experimental chest X-ray scoring system for quantifying and monitoring disease progression. La radiologia medica. 2020;125(5):509–13.
7. Borghesi A, Zigliani A, Golemi S, Carapella N, Maculotti P, Farina D, et al. Chest X-ray severity index as a predictor of in-hospital mortality in coronavirus disease 2019: A study of 302 patients from Italy. Int J Infect Dis. 2020;96:291–3.
8. Choi Y, Lee MK. Neuroimaging findings of brain MRI and CT in patients with COVID-19: A systematic review and meta-analysis. Eur J Radiol. 2020;133(109393):10939.
9. Francone M, Iafrate F, Masci G, Coco S, Cilia F, Manganaro L, et al. Chest CT score in COVID-19 patients: correlation with disease severity and short-term prognosis. European Radiology. 2020;30(12):6808–17.
10. Garg D, Muthu V, Sehgal IS, *et al.* Coronavirus Disease (COVID-19) Associated Mucormycosis (CAM): Case Report and Systematic Review of Literature. *Mycopathologia* Feb 2021, 289–98.
11. Garg M, Prabhakar N, Bhalla AS, Irodi A, Sehgal I, Debi U, Suri V, Agarwal R, Yaddanapudi LN, Puri GD, Sandhu MS. Computed tomography chest in COVID-19: When and why? Indian J Med Res. 2021 Jan and Feb;153(1 and 2):86–92.
12. Han X, Fan Y, Alwalid O, Li N, Jia X, Yuan M, et al. Six-month Follow-up Chest CT Findings after Severe COVID-19 Pneumonia. Radiology. 2021;299(1):E177–86.

13. Hani C, Trieu NH, Saab I, et al. COVID-19 pneumonia: A review of typical CT findings and differential diagnosis./*Diagn Interv Imaging*. 2020;101(5):263–8. doi:10.1016/j.diii.2020.03.014.

14. Kandemirli S, Dogan L, Sarikaya Z, Kara S, Akinci C, Kaya D, et al. Brain MRI Findings in Patients in the Intensive Care Unit with COVID-19 Infection. Radiology. 2020;297(1):E232–5.

15. Li K, Wu J, Wu F, Guo D, Chen L, Fang Z, et al. The Clinical and Chest CT Features Associated With Severe and Critical COVID-19 Pneumonia. Investigative Radiology. 2020;55(6):327–31.

16. Liu D, Zhang W, Pan F, Li L, Yang L, Zheng D, et al. The pulmonary sequelae in discharged patients with COVID-19: a short-term observational study. Respiratory Research. 2020;21(1).

17. Pan F, Ye T, Sun P, Gui S, Liang B, Li L, et al. Time Course of Lung Changes at Chest CT during Recovery from Coronavirus Disease 2019 (COVID-19). Radiology. 2020;295(3):715–21.

18. Penha D, Pinto EG, Matos F, Hochhegger B, Monaghan C, Taborda-Barata L, et al. CO-RADS: Coronavirus classification review. J Clin Imaging Sci. 2021;11(9):9.

19. Prokop M, van Everdingen W, van Rees Vellinga T, Quarles van Ufford H, Stöger L, Beenen L, et al. CO-RADS: A categorical CT assessment scheme for patients suspected of having COVID-19-definition and evaluation. Radiology. 2020;296(2):E97–104.

20. Revzin M, Raza S, Srivastava N, Warshawsky R, D'Agostino C, Malhotra A, et al. Multisystem Imaging Manifestations of COVID-19, Part 2: From Cardiac Complications to Pediatric Manifestations. RadioGraphics. 2020;40(7):1866–92.

21. Salehi S, Abedi A, Balakrishnan S, Gholamrezanezhad A. Coronavirus Disease 2019 (COVID-19): A Systematic Review of Imaging Findings in COVID-19 Patients./*AJR Am J Roentgenol*. 2020;215(1):87–93. doi:10.2214/AJR.20.23034

22. Tabatabaei SMH, Talari H, Gholamrezanezhad A, Farhood B, Rahimi H, Razzaghi R, et al. A low-dose chest CT protocol for the diagnosis of COVID-19 pneumonia: a prospective study. Emerg Radiol. 2020;27(6):607–15.

23. Thoracic Imaging in COVID-19 Infection. Guidance for the reporting radiologist. British Society of Thoracic Imaging. Version 2. 16th March 2020.

24. Tofighi S, Najafi S, Johnston SK, Gholamrezanezhad A. Low-dose CT in COVID-19 outbreak: radiation safety, image wisely, and image gently pledge. *Emerg Radiol*. 2020;27(6):601–5.

25. Yang R, Li X, Liu H, Zhen Y, Zhang X, Xiong Q, et al. Chest CT Severity Score: An Imaging Tool for Assessing Severe COVID-19. Radiology: Cardiothoracic Imaging. 2020;2(2):e200047.

Approach to Management

Suresh Kumar, Karan Chhabra

IDENTIFICATION AND MANAGEMENT OF COVID-19 PATIENTS

Case Definition

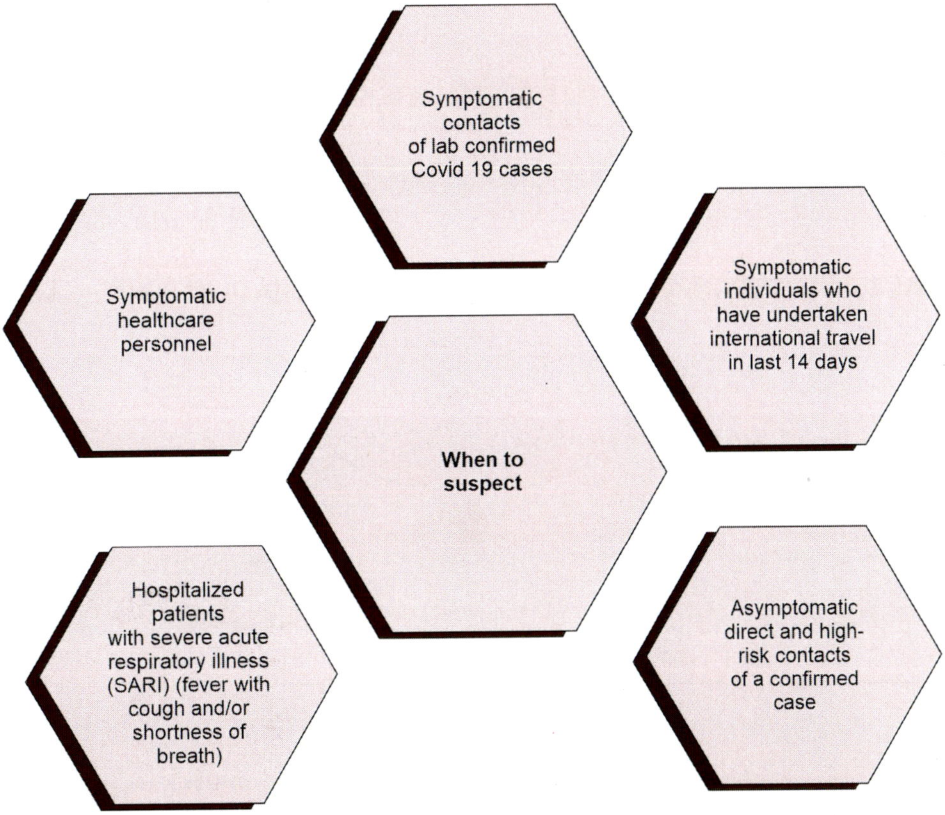

Symptomatic contacts of lab confirmed Covid 19 cases

Symptomatic individuals who have undertaken international travel in last 14 days

Symptomatic healthcare personnel

When to suspect

Hospitalized patients with severe acute respiratory illness (SARI) (fever with cough and/or shortness of breath)

Asymptomatic direct and high-risk contacts of a confirmed case

Who is a Confirmed Case?

Any person with laboratory confirmed COVID-19 infection, regardless of clinical signs and symptoms.

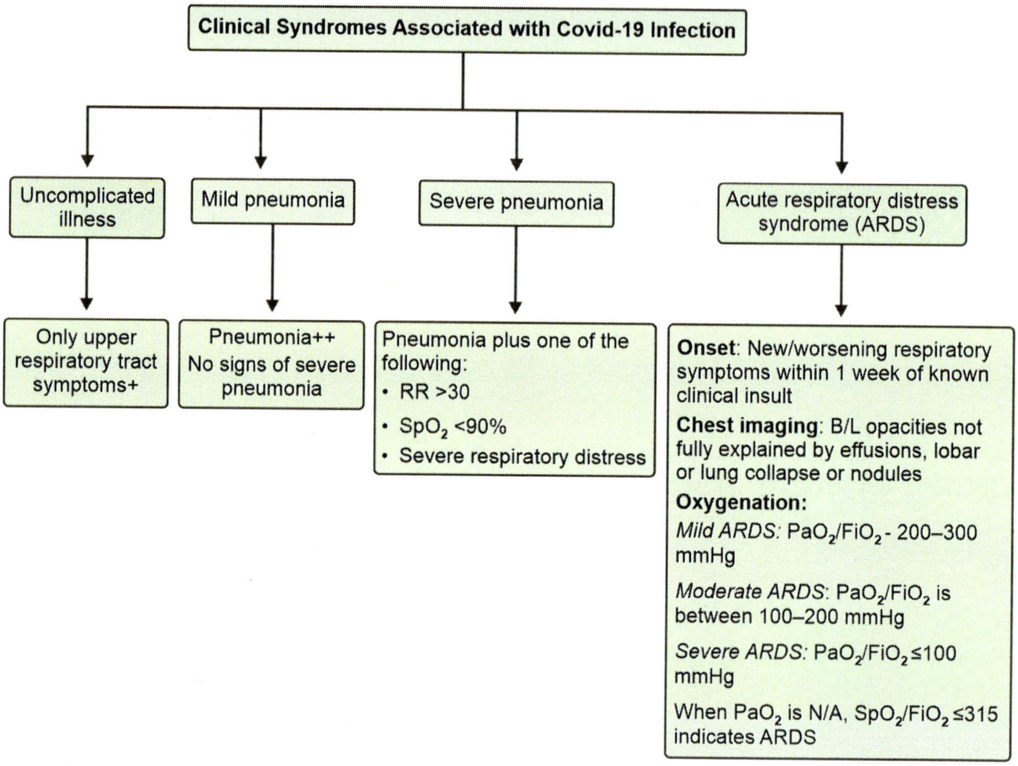

Clinical Syndromes Associated with Covid-19 Infection
Uncomplicated illness
Mild pneumonia
Severe pneumonia
Acute respiratory distress syndrome (ARDS)
Only upper respiratory tract symptoms+
Pneumonia++
No signs of severe pneumonia
Pneumonia plus one of the following:
• RR >30
• SpO_2 <90%
• Severe respiratory distress
Onset: New/worsening respiratory symptoms within 1 week of known clinical insult
Chest imaging: B/L opacities not fully explained by effusions, lobar or lung collapse or nodules
Oxygenation:
Mild ARDS: PaO_2/FiO_2 - 200–300 mmHg
Moderate ARDS: PaO_2/FiO_2 is between 100–200 mmHg
Severe ARDS: $PaO_2/FiO_2 \leq 100$ mmHg
When PaO_2 is N/A, $SpO_2/FiO_2 \leq 315$ indicates ARDS

PaO_2: Arterial partial pressure of O_2; FiO_2: Fraction of inspired oxygen; SpO_2: Oxygen saturation.

INITIAL SUPPORTIVE THERAPY OF ALL SUSPECTED COVID-19 PATIENTS

Start supplemental O_2 if SARI ++
Start @ 5l/min; target for $SpO_2 \geq 90\%$
Conservative
Fluid management
Care of comorbidities (HTN, DM, CAD, COPD, CKD)
Supportive therapy
Early initiation of empirical antibiotics (if sepsis++)
Give corticosteroids in case of moderate to severe case

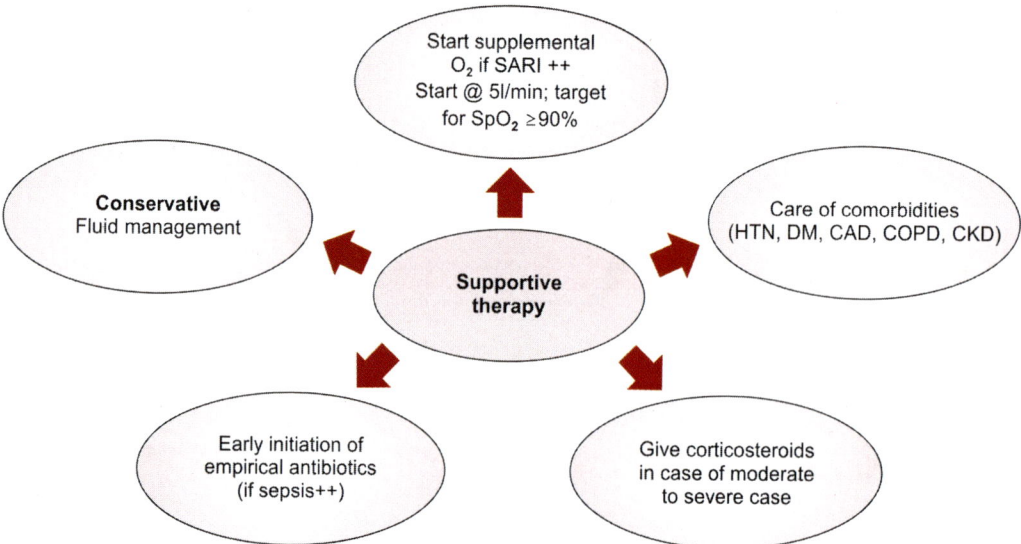

SARI: Severe acute respiratory illness; HTN: Hypertension; DM: Diabetes mellitus; CAD: Coronary artery disease; COPD: Chronic obstructive pulmonary disease; CKD: Chronic kidney disease.

MANAGEMENT OF MILD CASE OF COVID-19

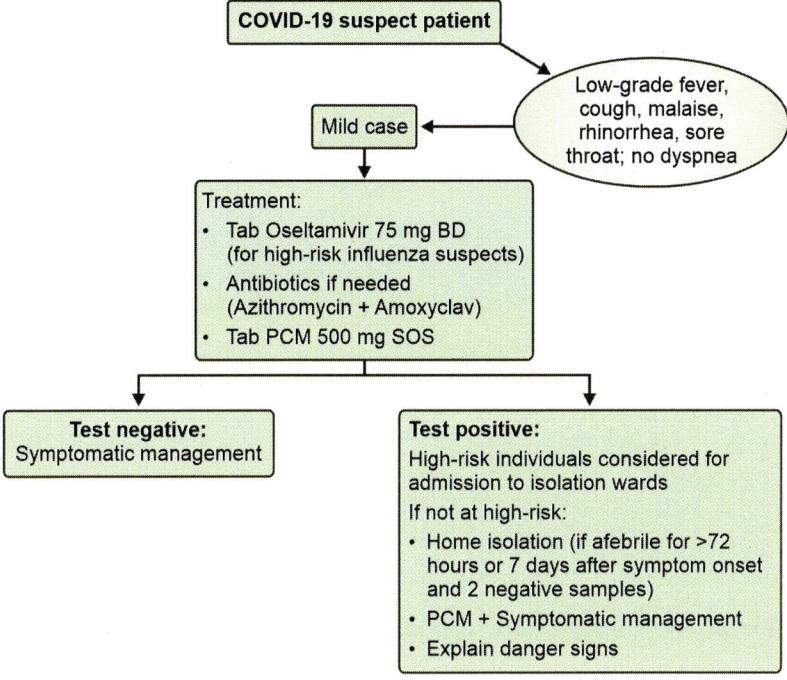

COVID-19 suspect patient

Low-grade fever, cough, malaise, rhinorrhea, sore throat; no dyspnea

Mild case

Treatment:
- Tab Oseltamivir 75 mg BD (for high-risk influenza suspects)
- Antibiotics if needed (Azithromycin + Amoxyclav)
- Tab PCM 500 mg SOS

Test negative: Symptomatic management

Test positive:
High-risk individuals considered for admission to isolation wards
If not at high-risk:
- Home isolation (if afebrile for >72 hours or 7 days after symptom onset and 2 negative samples)
- PCM + Symptomatic management
- Explain danger signs

MANAGEMENT OF MODERATE CASE

Moderate case: Pneumonia with no signs of severe disease
RR $\geq$24/min OR SpO$_2$ <94% on room air

Oxygen support:
- Target SpO$_2$: 92–96% (88–92% in case of COPD)
- Preferred device for oxygenation: Non-rebreathing face mask
- Awake proning may be used in patients with persistent hypoxemia despite oxygen >4L/min.

Anticoagulation:
Prophylactic dose of LMWH/UFH, if not contraindicated (enoxaparin 40 mg daily SC)

Corticosteroids:
IV Methylprednisolone 0.5–1.0 mg/kg OR
Dexamethasone 0.1–0.2 mg/kg for 3–5 days

Antivirals:
Tab HCQS 400 mg BD on Day 1 followed by 400 mg OD × 4 days (after assessment of ECG for QT interval)

Investigational therapies:
1. Inj Remdisvir 200 mg IV on day 1 followed by 100 mg IV daily for next 4 days (total 5 day therapy)
2. Inj Tocilizumab 8 mg/kg (max dose 800 mg once; usual dose 400 mg; dose can be repeated after 12–24 hours if no improvement occurs with the first dose
3. Convalescent plasma (200 ml single dose, may be repeated 24 hours later)

MANAGEMENT OF SEVERE CASE

Severe case

Oxygenation:
- If work of breathing is low: Trial of CPAP with oronasal mask/NIV with helmet interface/HFNC
- If work of breathing is high/Not tolerating NIV: Consider Intubation

Anticoagulation:
High dose prophylactic dose of LMWH/UFH, if not contraindicated (enoxaparin 40 mg or 0.5 mg/kg BD SC)

Corticosteroids:
IV Methylprednisolone 1–2 mg/kg OR
Dexamethasone 0.2–0.4 mg/kg for 5–7 days

Investigational therapies:
1. Inj Remdisvir 200 mg IV on day 1 followed by 100 mg IV daily for next 4 days (total 5 day therapy)
2. Inj Tocilizumab 8 mg/kg (max dose 800 mg once; usual dose 400 mg; dose can be repeated after 12–24 hours if no improvement occurs with the first dose
3. Convalescent plasma (200 ml single dose, may be repeated 24 hours later)

RR: Respiratory rate; SBP: Systolic blood pressure; DBP: Diastolic blood pressure; MDIs: Metered dose inhalers; HCQ: Hydroxychloroquine; MODS: *Multiple organ dysfunction syndrome; ICU: Intensive care unit;* NIV: Noninvasive ventilation; HFNC: *High-flow nasal cannula;* ARDS: Acute respiratory distress syndrome; HME: Heat and moisture exchanger; ECMO: *Extracorporeal membrane oxygenation.*

MANAGEMENT OF ARDS IN PATIENT OF COVID

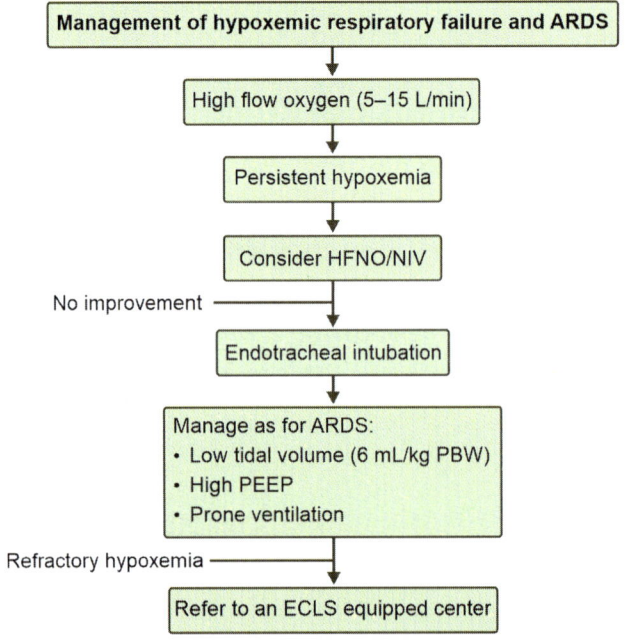

ARDS: Acute respiratory distress syndrome; HFNO: High frequency nasal oxygenation; NIV: Non-invasive ventilation; PEEP: Positive end-expiratory pressure; ECLS: Extracorporeal life support.

MANAGEMENT OF SEPSIS AND SEPTIC SHOCK IN COVID-19 PATIENTS

Definitions

Sepsis: Life-threatening organ dysfunction occurring as a result of a dysregulated host response to suspected or proven infection, with organ dysfunction. Signs of organ dysfunction include altered mental status, difficult or fast breathing, low oxygen saturation, reduced urine output, fast heart rate, weak pulse, cold extremities or low blood pressure, skin mottling, or laboratory evidence of coagulopathy, thrombocytopenia, acidosis, high lactate or hyperbilirubinemia.

Septic shock refers to persisting hypotension despite volume resuscitation, requiring vasopressors to maintain mean arterial pressure (MAP) ≥65 mmHg and serum lactate level >2 mmol/L.

Pearls in management of septic shock:
- 30 mL/kg of isotonic crystalloids in the first 3 hours.
- Start antibiotics within the 1st hour of recognition of septic shock.
- Perfusion targets: MAP >65 mmHg; Urine output >0.5 ml/kg/hour; improvement in skin mottling, capillary refill, level of consciousness and serum lactate.
- Administer vasopressors when shock persists during or after fluid resuscitation. The initial blood pressure target is MAP ≥65 mmHg.

Points to be Noted
- **Norepinephrine** is recommended as first choice of vasopressor.
- **Vasopressin** should be used with the intent of reducing the dose of norepinephrine.
- Use of **dopamine is to be avoided.**
- Dobutamine use is suggested when patients show evidence of hypoperfusion despite adequate fluid loading and use of vasopressors.

Intensive Care Management of Critically Ill COVID-19 Patients

Suresh Kumar, Lalita Chaudhary

The ongoing COVID-19 pandemic have overwhelmed the healthcare capacity of the affected regions all over the world. Italy, a high-income country with 12.5 critical care beds per 100000 population, continues to struggle with the outbreak. China, an upper-middle-income country, has 3.6 critical care beds per 100000 population, and Wuhan was initially overwhelmed by COVID-19. In United States, over one-third of cases having to wait 6 hours or more for transfer to ICU. As the ICU capacity across the globe is strained and more than 80% cases of COVID-19 have mild form of disease, it is vital to timely identify moderate to severe cases of COVID-19 which might benefit from ICU admission.

CRITERIA FOR ADMISSION TO ICU

An early warning score (EWS) is a simple, reproducible score, calculated at the bedside, to identify patients who are, or are at risk of becoming, critically ill. The score is a modified version of the national early warning score (NEWS) with age ≥65 years added as an independent risk factor based on recent reports (Table 8.1).

TABLE 8.1: Early warning score (EWS)							
Parameter	3	2	1	0	1	2	3
Age (years)				<65			≤65
Respiratory rate (per minute)	≤8		9–11	12–20		21–24	≤25
Oxygen saturation in room air (%)	≤91	92–93	94–95	≥96			
Any oxygen supplementation		Yes		No			
Pulse (per minute)	≤40		41–50	51–90	91–110	111–130	≥131
Systolic BP (mmHg)	≤90	91–100	101–110	111–219			≥220
Consciousness				Alert			Drowsiness Lethargy Coma Confusion
Temperature (°C)	≤35.0		35.1–36	36.1–38	38.1–39	≥39.1	

Based on scores of EWS, following decision regarding management of COVID-19 patients can be considered;
- 04 points: Hospitalization without special additional supervision.
- 56 points (or ≥3 points in one parameter): Intermediate care unit (IMCU) or monitoring unit/room.
- >6 points: Intensive care unit (ICU).

OUTCOME OF COVID-19 CASES ADMITTED IN ICU

Initial reports from China, Italy and United States suggest high mortality rate with case fatality rate of around 50%. Majority of cases were admitted in ICU due to hypoxemic respiratory failure and some of them had concurrent hypotension requiring vasopressors.

In view of these findings we here discuss the ICU management of COVID-19 patients requiring respiratory support and management of hypotension.

RESPIRATORY SUPPORT FOR PATIENTS WITH COVID-19

COVID-19 mainly affects respiratory system with some patients rapidly progressing to acute respiratory distress syndrome (ARDS); other organ functions are less commonly affected. The patients with moderate or severe involvement of respiratory system are likely to be admitted in ICU for respiratory support and are at risk of death. The elderly and those with comorbidities are at highest risk of mortality.

RECOMMENDATION FOR OXYGEN SUPPLEMENTATION IN COVID-19

In adult patients with COVID-19, it is recommended to start oxygen supplementation if SpO_2 is less than 90%. As hyperoxia is associated with potential patient harm, SpO_2 should be maintained no higher than 96%.

Devices for Oxygen Supplementation

For management of COVID-19 associated respiratory failure, full spectrum of invasive and noninvasive options must be considered. A number of noninvasive respiratory support options exit to support COVID-19 patients with mild to moderate respiratory distress. However, all forms of supplemental oxygenation and respiratory support have potential to aerosolize respiratory pathogens. Selection of respiratory support therefore must balance between clinical benefit against risks of nosocomial infection. The exhaled air dispersion distance of various oxygen delivery devices is shown in Table 8.2.

As non-rebreathing mask has least dispersion of exhaled air, it should be preferred over other oxygen delivery devices in COVID-19 patients with respiratory failure.

High Flow Nasal Cannula (HFNC)

In patients with acute hypoxemic respiratory failure, HFNC has been proven to avoid intubation compared to conventional oxygen device. However, there is an important concern that HFNC may increase bio-aerosol dispersion due to the high gas flow used. This concern is reflected in the limited use of HFNC in the early clinical reports of COVID-19. The scientific evidence of generation and dispersion of bio-aerosols *via*

TABLE 8.2: Maximum exhaled air dispersion during various oxygen delivery devices

Oxygen delivery devices	Oxygen flow (L/min)	Maximum exhaled air dispersion distance(m)		
Nasal cannula	1	0.30		
	3	0.36		
	5	0.45		
Simple face mask	4	0.20		
	6	0.22		
	8	0.30		
	10	0.40, >0.40 during cough		
Venturi mask	24% FiO_2	*Normal lungs*	*Severe lung injury*	
		0.4	0.32	
	40% FiO_2	0.33	0.29	
Non rebreathing mask	6, 8, 10, 12	<0.1		
Jet nebulization	6	*Normal lungs*	*Mild lung injury*	*Severe lung injury*
		0.45	0.54	>0.80
Noninvasive ventilation	Depending on type of mask and inspiratory and expiratory pressures	0.40 to > 0.95 m		

HFNC have showed a similar risk to standard oxygen masks. Therefore, application of HFNC with a surgical mask on patient's face above could thus be a reasonable practice in hypoxemic COVID-19 patients to avoid intubation and mechanical ventilation.

Based on above discussion, following algorithm is suggested for management of COVID-19 with respiratory failure (Fig. 8.1).

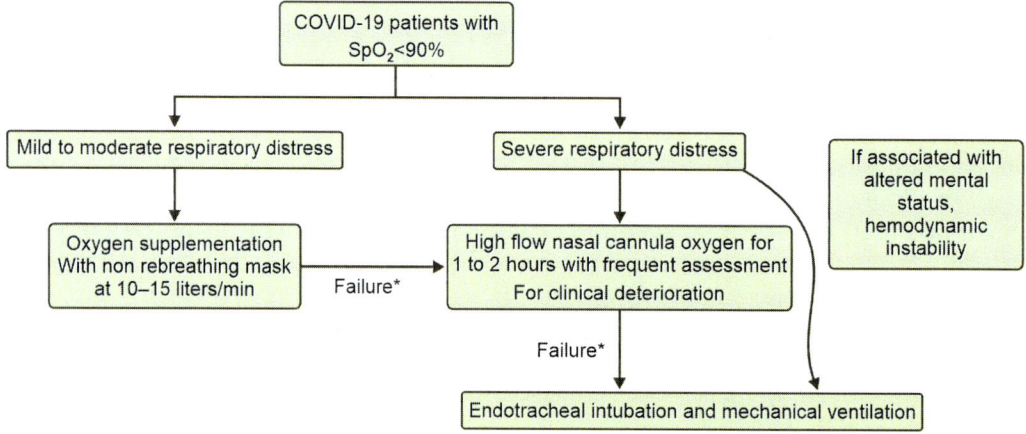

*Increasing respiratory distress and failure to maintain SpO_2 <90%

Fig. 8.1: Algorithm for COVID-19 patients with respiratory failure

Noninvasive Ventilation (NIV)

It is provided as CPAP via nasal canula or oronasal mask or as NIV via helmets or full-face mask. NIV is not routinely recommended for management of hypoxemic respiratory failure of SARS-CoV-2 as it is associated with high failure rate, delayed intubation and increased risk of aerosol exposure due to poor fit of mask. It may temporarily improve oxygenation and reduce work of breathing in patients of COVID-19 with respiratory failure but does not alter the natural course of viral pneumonia. In a clinical report from Italy, NIV was used for a specific cohort of patients; those in early phase of COVID 19 with hypercapnic respiratory failure such as those with COPD. They recommended a single attempt of 1 hour with NIV and if no substantial improvement is observed early endotracheal intubation and mechanical ventilation should be considered.

Invasive Mechanical Ventilation

Mechanically ventilated patients with COVID-19 should be managed similar to other patients of ALI/ARDS. While mechanical ventilation is life saving in these patients it can worsen lung injury through ventilator induced lung injury. Therefore, it is strongly recommended to use low tidal volume ventilation targeting plateau pressure (Pplat <30 cm H_2O) as per ARDS Net Study Protocol (Fig. 8.2).

For patients with moderate to severe ARDS, it has been suggested to use higher PEEP (>10 cm H_2O) with close monitoring for risk of barotrauma. Application of extrinsic PEEP prevents repeated opening and closing of alveoli, i.e. atelectotrauma and hence VILI. It also improves oxygenation by improved and sustained alveolar recruitment.

For patients on MV, prone positioning for 12 to 16 hours per day has been suggested as radiological feature of lungs from initial predominant pattern of ground glass opacities progressed to mixed pattern with predominant basilar consolidation in COVID-19. Prone positioning improves oxygenation by reducing the ventral and dorsal transpulmonary pressure, reducing lung compression and improving perfusion. To facilitate protective lung ventilation intermittent boluses of neuromuscular blockers should be used. Continuous infusion of NMB for up to 48 hours is recommended if there is persistent ventilator dyssynchrony, persistently high plateau pressure, for prone positioning or if there is need for deep sedation.

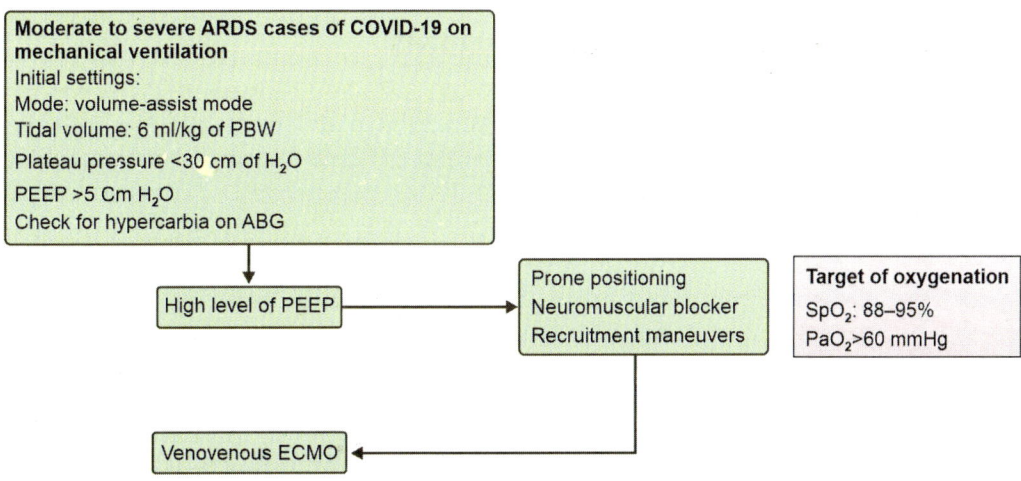

Fig. 8.2: Mechanical ventilation strategy in COVID-19

Despite optimizing ventilation if there is refractory hypoxemia, recruitment maneuvers can be utilized to open atelectatic alveoli. If facilities for ECMO is available, in carefully selected patients with COVID-19 and severe ARDS, venovenous ECMO is recommended.

HEMODYNAMIC SUPPORT IN COVID-19 CASES

COVID-19 infection can lead to exacerbation of pre-existing cardiovascular conditions and also lead to cardiovascular complications, such as myocarditis, myocardial injury, acute coronary syndrome, cardiac arrhythmias and heart failure. These complications can lead to shock in patients admitted in ICU.

Risk factors associated with development of shock are older age, comorbidities especially diabetes and cardiac disease, lower lymphocyte count, higher D-dimer levels and possibly cardiac injury.

In acute treatment of shock conservative over liberal fluid therapy has been recommended based on fluid responsiveness of patient. To assess fluid responsiveness dynamic parameters, such as skin temperature, capillary refilling time and/or serum lactate measurement has been recommended over static parameters, such as CVP or mean arterial pressure measurement. In mechanically ventilated patient dynamic parameters with higher accuracy, such as passive leg raise, pulse pressure variation or stroke volume variation can be used.

For management of shock, buffered/balanced crystalloids are preferred over colloids. The first line vasoactive agent for shock in COVID-19 associated shock is norepinephrine. If norepinephrine is not available, either epinephrine or vasopressin has been suggested over other vasoactive drugs. The target MAP for titration of vasoactive drugs are 60–65 mmHg.

If there is evidence of cardiac dysfunction in patients and despite fluid resuscitation and norepinephrine there is persistent hypoperfusion, dobutamine can be added to improve circulation. For refractory hypotension low dose corticosteroid therapy ("shock-reversal") can be considered.

HYPERCOAGULABILITY IN CRITICALLY ILL PATIENTS

COVID-19 infection may predispose patients to thrombotic disease, both in the venous and arterial circulations, due to excessive inflammation, platelet activation, endothelial dysfunction, and stasis. The coagulation anomaly is characterized by increase in procoagulant factor levels including increase in fibrinogen and D-dimers that have been linked with high mortality. In patients with severe disease both disseminated intravascular coagulopathy and sepsis induced coagulopathy have been reported.

Based on these findings it is vital to start on prophylactic anticoagulation in the absence of an absolute contraindication. As the standard thromboprophylaxis in ICU have failure rate of 5–10% and clinical progression of COVID-19 infection is unpredictable, some experts suggested that therapeutic anticoagulation might have preventive role in development of microvascular thrombosis. The French guidance document recommends full-dose therapeutic dose anticoagulation for patients with increased fibrinogen >8 g/dl or D-dimer >3.0 µg/ml.

Connor et al advocated a risk adapted approach to escalating dose of anticoagulation after assessing the bleeding risk of each patient with monitoring of fibrinogen, PT, aPTT and renal functions.

STRESS-ULCER PROPHYLAXIS

Critically ill patients in ICU are at increased risk of stress related gastrointestinal bleed. However, the routine administration of stress ulcer prophylaxis is not recommended in ICU as it increases the risk for ventilator associated pneumonia and increases patient mortality. SUP should be administered to patients who are at very high-risk or high-risk of GI bleed such as those with coagulopathy, on prolonged mechanical ventilation (>48 hours), sepsis, hypotension, etc.

NUTRITION IN COVID-19 ICU PATIENTS

Patients of COVID-19 admitted to ICU are at high nutritional risk due to the underlying medical condition and medical management strategies such as early mechanical ventilation, deep sedation, prone positioning and conservative fluid approach. Alteration in metabolism, and gastrointestinal function, coupled with nutritional deficits during critical illness and following, are all likely to contribute to a decline in nutrition status and poorer functional ability. The nutritional guidelines for COVID-19 patients in ICU recommends following main points:

1. Provision of early enteral nutrition.
2. Aim for daily caloric intake of 20–25 kCal/kg/day; hypocaloric (70% of recommended) nutrition is advised in the first 3–7 days with commencement with 24–48 hours. Based on tolerance of patient calorie intake should be gradually increased.
3. Daily protein delivery of at least 1.2 g/kg/day.
4. Monitoring of gastric residual volume (GRV) to prevent risk of vomiting and aspiration, a lower GRV of <300 ml is recommended by British and Australian/ New Zealand guidelines.

Infection Prevention and Control

Sandeep Garg, Vikas Manchanda, Pradeep Kumar

At point of triage/first contact

- Give the **suspect patient** a triple layer surgical mask
- Keep ≥1 meter **distance** between suspected patients
- Instruct all patients to **cover nose and mouth** during coughing/sneezing

Droplet precautions

- Use triple layer surgical **masks** if working within 1–2 meters of the patient
- Place patients in **single rooms**, or group together those with the same etiological diagnosis
- Use **eye protection** if working in contact with patients with respiratory symptoms

Contact precautions

- Use PPE in patient isolation rooms
- Use dedicated equipment (stethoscopes/BP cuffs)
- Hand hygiene
- Ensure adequate ventilation

Airborne precautions when performing aerosol generating procedures (intubation/CPR/suctioning/bronchoscopy)

- Use PPE during such procedures
- Negative pressure rooms

THE SEVEN STEPS OF EFFECTIVE HANDWASHING

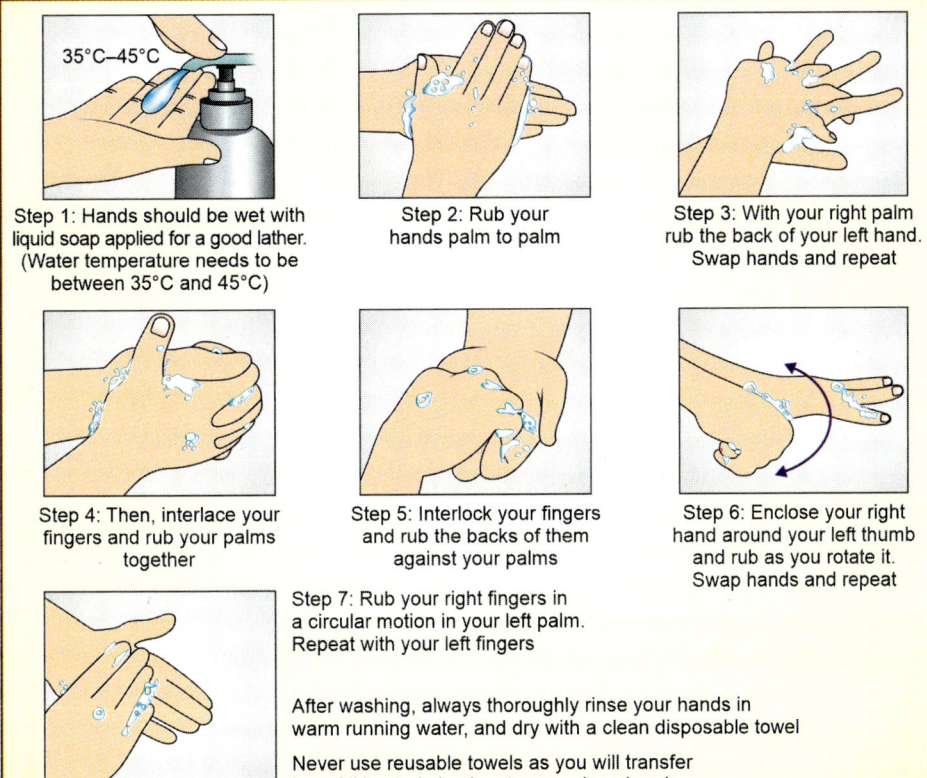

(*Source:* https://www.highspeedtraining.co.uk/hub/7-steps-of-hand-washing-poster/)

GENERAL SOCIAL PREVENTIVE MEASURES TO CONTROL INFECTION

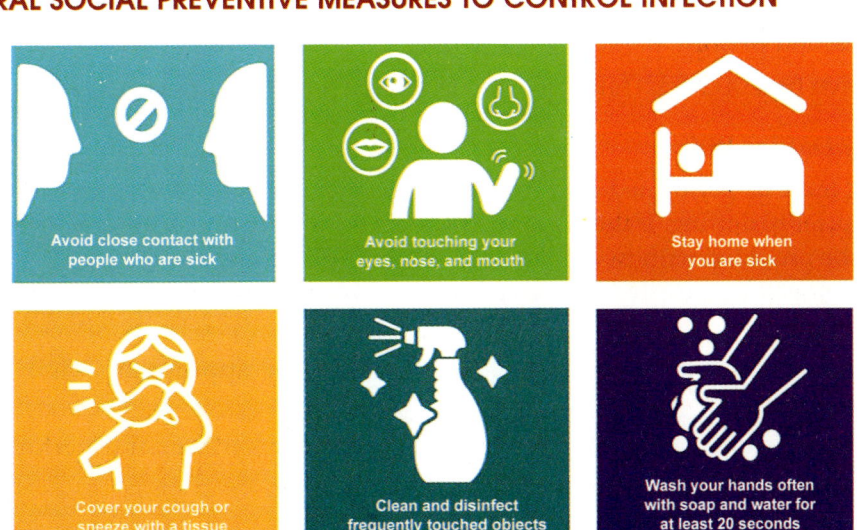

(*Source:* https://www.gillettechildrens.org/khm/covid-19-what-you-need-to-know)

PREVENTIVE MEASURES FOR HEALTHCARE WORKERS

Steps of Donning PPE (Steps may vary depending on the kit used):

Donning of the PPE must be performed in designated area.

1. Remove home clothes, jewelry, watches, electronic gadgets, etc. and don clean hospital scrubs.
2. Wash hands with soap and water.
3. Wear shoe covers; tie lace in front of the shin.
4. Wear first set of gloves; it should be smaller than second pair, of comfortable size, can be sterile or unsterile.
5. Wear a clean disposable nonpermeable gown; sleeves of gown should cover the gloves at the wrists, tie the lace behind snuggly without wrapping all around the waist. Decontaminate the gown if it becomes soiled. Remove gown only in designated doffing area and discard the gown (yellow bin) before leaving patient care area.
6. Wear the N-95 respirator by cupping the mask in hand, placing the lower strap behind the neck passing below ears, and then placing the upper strap over back of head passing above ears. Check for snug fit of mask. There should be no more than minimal air leak from sides.
7. Wear eyepiece by adjusting the strap according to required size. Open the ports at upper end to prevent fogging while wearing; upper end of N-95 mask should be covered by eyepiece.
8. Wear the hood which should lay over the gown without leaving any open space.
9. Wear second pair of gloves. They should be of larger size than first pair, should cover free end of arms of gown. Change gloves if they become torn or contaminated. Remove and discard gloves while leaving the patient room or care area, and perform hand hygiene at once.
10. Gown fitness check: Take help of companion for fitness check.

Steps of Doffing PPE

Doffing must be performed only in the designated area; check for any leak or soiling in PPE prior to doffing. If there is any, disinfect the area before doffing. Doffing room should be provided with two chairs, one labeled "dirty" and the other as "clean". All the PPE must be discarded in the yellow bin. Hand hygiene is essential after every step.

1. Disinfect the hands wearing gloves by following appropriate hand hygiene procedure.
2. Remove shoe covers only by touching the outer surface, and perform hand hygiene.
3. Remove outer gloves and perform hand hygiene.
4. Remove hood and perform hand hygiene.

5. Remove the gown slowly by holding it at the waist and pullling. Without touching the outer surface, remove it with a rolling inside out technique. Perform hand hygiene.

6. Remove eyepiece by holding the straps, and perform hand hygiene.

7. Remove inner gloves and perform hand hygiene.

8. Wear another pair of sterile/unsterile gloves.

9. Remove mask. Be careful not to touch the exposed surface of mask. First remove lower strap of mask, then remove the mask holding upper strap in a slow and steady pace (as to not generate aerosols).

10. Perform hand hygiene.

11. Sit over clean chair and clean your shoes with alcohol swabs.

12. Remove last pair of gloves and perform hand hygiene.

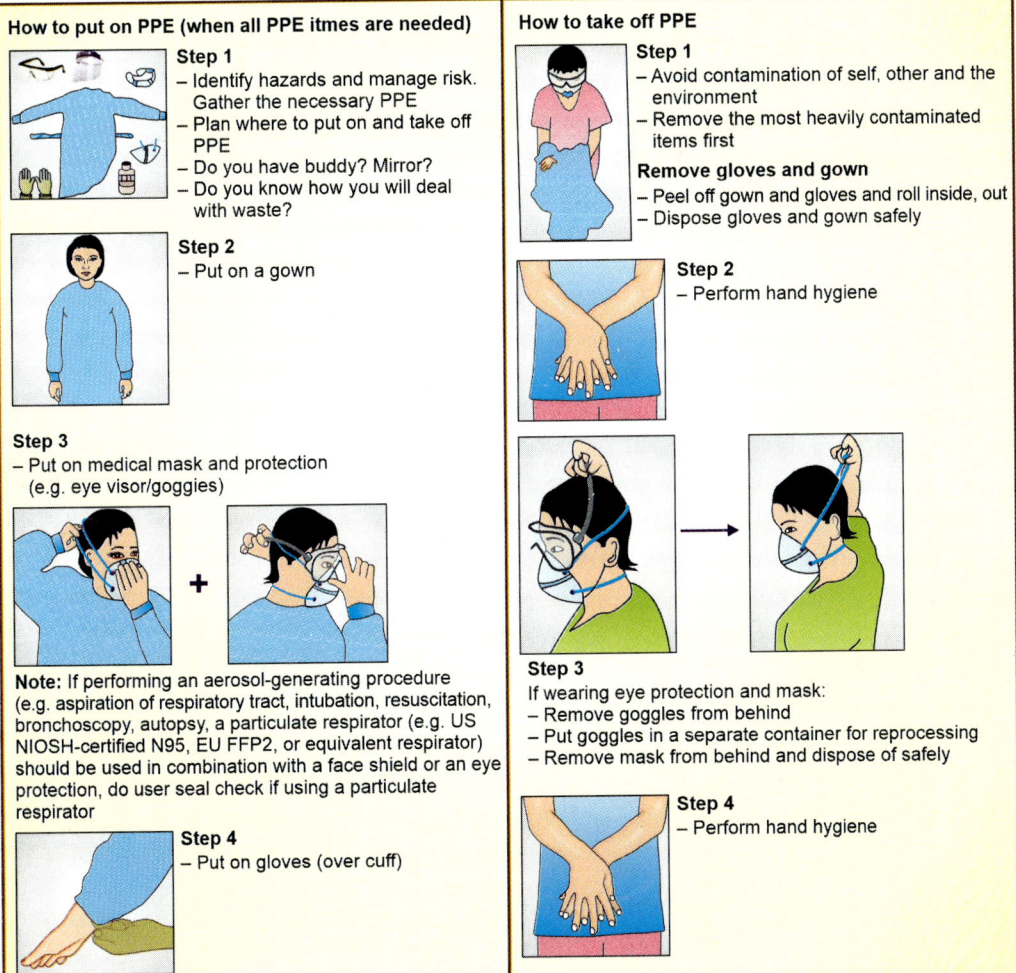

How to put on PPE (when all PPE itmes are needed)

Step 1
– Identify hazards and manage risk. Gather the necessary PPE
– Plan where to put on and take off PPE
– Do you have buddy? Mirror?
– Do you know how you will deal with waste?

Step 2
– Put on a gown

Step 3
– Put on medical mask and protection (e.g. eye visor/goggies)

+

Note: If performing an aerosol-generating procedure (e.g. aspiration of respiratory tract, intubation, resuscitation, bronchoscopy, autopsy, a particulate respirator (e.g. US NIOSH-certified N95, EU FFP2, or equivalent respirator) should be used in combination with a face shield or an eye protection, do user seal check if using a particulate respirator

Step 4
– Put on gloves (over cuff)

How to take off PPE

Step 1
– Avoid contamination of self, other and the environment
– Remove the most heavily contaminated items first

Remove gloves and gown
– Peel off gown and gloves and roll inside, out
– Dispose gloves and gown safely

Step 2
– Perform hand hygiene

Step 3
If wearing eye protection and mask:
– Remove goggles from behind
– Put goggles in a separate container for reprocessing
– Remove mask from behind and dispose of safely

Step 4
– Perform hand hygiene

Estimated role of preventive measures in limiting the spread of COVID-19

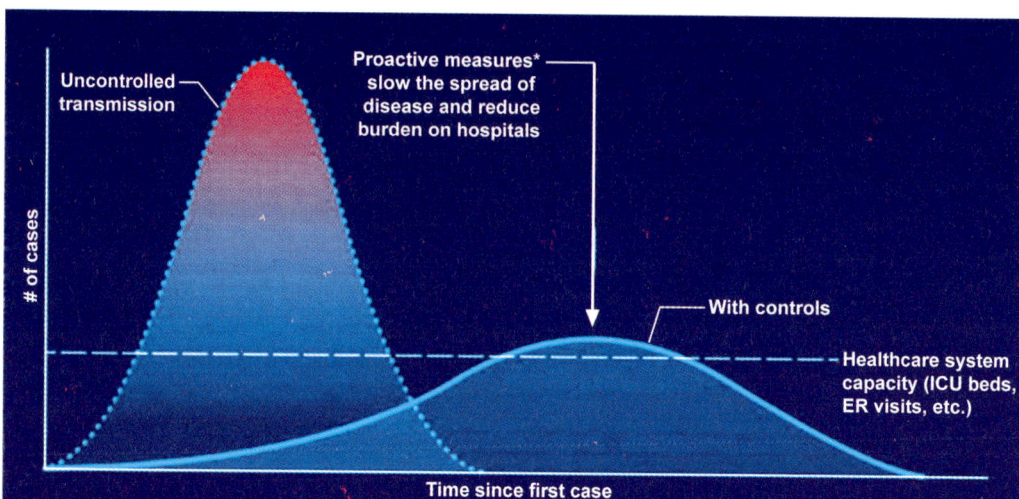

Source: http://ctbergstrom.com/covid19.html (wikimedia commons)

ICMR PREVENTIVE MEASURES TO BE TAKEN TO CONTAIN THE SPREAD OF NOVEL CORONAVIRUS (COVID-19)

Measures which should be followed by everyone:

1. Maintaining personal hygiene and social distancing.
2. Practicing frequent handwashing and washing hands with soap and water or using alcohol-based hand rub.
3. Covering nose and mouth with handkerchief or tissue while sneezing or coughing.
4. Throwing used tissues into closed bins immediately after use.
5. Maintaining a safe distance from people during interaction, especially with those having flu-like symptoms.
6. Sneezing into the inner side of your elbow.
7. Charting temperature regularly and checking for respiratory symptoms.
8. Consulting a doctor if respiratory symptoms persist.
9. While visiting a doctor, wear a mask/cloth to cover mouth and nose.

Things which should not be done:

1. Shake hands.
2. Touch your eyes, nose and mouth unnecessarily.
3. Sneeze or cough into palms of your hands.
4. Spit in public.
5. Travel unnecessarily, particularly to any affected region.
6. Participate in large gatherings, including sitting in groups at canteens.
7. Visit gyms, clubs and crowded places.

The 5T Plan to Tackle COVID-19

The Delhi Government has taken up a huge initiative to counter this pandemic.

1. **Testing:** The Government plans robust testing for COVID-19 amongst contacts of positive patients as well as in hotspot areas such as religious congregations.

2. **Tracing:** Contact tracing is an essential part of containing epidemics. All people who have potentially come in contact with COVID-19 positive patients will be traced and be asked to remain in strict self-quarantine. Help of the police authorities will be taken to ensure tracing and subsequent quarantine.

3. **Treatment:** The Government has earmarked certain hospitals that will purely cater to COVID affected patients. Hotel rooms will be used for the purpose of quarantine.

4. **Teamwork:** Will require coordination between Center and State Governments, Public and Private Sector.

5. **Tracking and monitoring:** To ensure containment of this unprecedented epidemic, there needs to be appropriate monitoring of efficacy of the above-mentioned measures. This will help point out the pitfalls in management and to redirect resources in those areas.

Surgery in COVID Times

Rajdeep Singh, Lovenish Bains

The second wave of COVID-19 in Delhi overwhelmed available resources, and elective surgical cases took a back seat so as to concentrate all manpower for critical COVID patients. The medical community now has more knowledge of how the infection spreads, and the data can be extrapolated for surgical procedures also.

With the decline in cases, many people have become lax with precautions, which can lead to another resurgence (3rd wave) whereas the dominant delta strain is said to be more infective and lethal. The following provides a practice guideline for the surgeon.

SPREAD OF INFECTION

Evidence is now in favor of airborne spread instead of droplet infection and fomites. This implies that a single patient in a general ward can infect multiple persons. Similarly, an infected patient reporting to OPD can be responsible for transmitting disease to many other patients. For the surgeons, it may be important to know that SARS-CoV-2 RNA has also been detected in other biological samples, including the urine and feces of some patient. However, there have been no published reports of transmission of SARS-CoV-2 through feces or urine. Some studies have also reported detection of SARS-CoV-2 RNA, in either plasma or serum, and the virus can replicate in blood cells. However, the role of bloodborne transmission remains uncertain; and low viral titres in plasma and serum suggest that the risk of transmission through this route may be low.

The single most effective preventive measure is to ensure masks are worn by all. Ideally an N95 mask should be worn; simple surgical masks may be used if N95 are not available. Hand disinfection should still be practised since it is an important route of spread of infection.

OUT PATIENT DEPARTMENT

The main strategy in any hospital should be to avoid unnecessary crowding in all its areas including out patient department (OPD), wards, and operating rooms (ORs). It would be ideal to test all patients and relatives for COVID-19 before coming to the hospital; however this is not a practical solution especially in a hospital like Lok Nayak Hospital where daily OPD attendance can exceed 3,000 persons.

Screening patients for symptoms and selective testing is more feasible. All persons coming to the OPDs should be screened for fever and asked about vaccination and history of COVID infection. Suspects should undergo RAT or TrueNAT testing for rapid reports. Positive cases may be referred to COVID clinic for appropriate advice.

At the same time, needy persons should not be deprived of medical care just because they are COVID positive or have a recent history of this infection.

TESTING

There are three main antigen tests available:
a. RT-PCR is currently the gold standard. Procedures which involve aerosol generation in relation to respiratory tract should ideally have a negative RT-PCR test. This includes tracheal intubation for anesthesia, bronchoscopy, endoscopy, endoscopic ENT procedures, etc. It is not required for procedures done under local anesthesia.
b. RAT (**rapid** antigen test): A good screening tool, but sensitivity is low for its routine use preoperatively.
c. TrueNat: Newer automated TrueNAT kits detect RdRp gene which can be used in place of RT-PCR for confirmation of diagnosis. It can replace RT-PCR testing, especially in places where RT-PCR testing facilities are not available.

RISK STRATIFICATION

A risk stratification/triage proposed by *Inter Association surgical practice recommendations in COVID 19era, Elective Surgery Acuity Scale (ESAS) developed by American College of Surgeons* or *Prioritization criteria for elective surgery during COVID 19 pandemic by NHS* can be utilized for triage of surgical procedures (Table 10.1). These are largely applicable during the pandemic peaks and not applicable when the positivity rate is under control.

TABLE 10.1: Triage for surgery during COVID 19 pandemic

Guidelines	Priority	Definition	Action
Inter association surgical practice recommendations	Emergency life-threatening conditions	Those conditions in which immediate surgical intervention is required and there is not enough time available to do and get the results of COVID 19 testing, e.g. life-threatening traumatic hemoperitoneum with hemodynamic instability, bowel gangrene.	Immediate (within hours)
	Emergency procedures	Those procedures that require immediate surgical intervention but provide a window of few hours to get COVID 19 testing. Interim non-surgical intervention could also be an option, e.g. bowel obstruction, perforation of hollow viscus, unresolved obstruction, complicated appendicitis, complicated cholecystitis.	Early (within 24–48 hours)
	Semi-emergent procedures	These includes condition where the procedure can be deferred for a few weeks or months but not more than 3 months due to worsening of symptoms or progression of stage of disease affecting final outcome, e.g. major malignancies.	Defer (but not more than 3 months)

(Contd.)

TABLE 10.1: Triage for surgery during COVID 19 pandemic (Contd.)

Guidelines	Priority	Definition	Action
	Elective procedures	These include those procedures which can be postponed by 3 months or more with mutual consent between patient and surgeon with no untoward effect on final outcome, e.g. uncomplicated groin hernia, varicose veins	Postpone
National health service [9B]	Level 1a/1b	1a: Emergency operation (<24 h) 1b: Urgent operation (<72 h)	Do not postpone
	Level 2	Deferrable for up to 4 weeks: • Cancer according to MDT decision • Crohn's disease-related complications • Goiter (mild moderate stridor) • Medically resistant thyrotoxicosis/ hyperparathyroidism/adrenal pathology	Balance the risk from the under-underlying condition with the need of viral containment to maximize safety
	Level 3	Deferrable for up to 3 months: • Cancer according to MDT decision • Cholecystectomy post-acute pancreatitis • Hernia presenting with complications • Parathyroidectomy—with medically resistant complications	Postpone
	Level 4	Deferrable beyond 3 months: • Uncomplicated hernias (hiatal, incisional) • Stomas closure included Hartmann's reversal • Proctology procedures • Upper UGI benign conditions (e.g gall-stones. MRGE, others) • Benign uncomplicated endocrine diseases • Breast reconstruction/prophylactic surgery/ benign diseases	Postpone
American College of Surgeons [9A]	Tier 1a	Low acuity surgery/healthy patient; (Out-patient surgery; Not life-threatening illness)	Postpone surgery or perform at ASC
	Tier 1b	Low acuity surgery/unhealthy patient	Postpone surgery or perform at ASC
	Tier 2a	Intermediate acuity surgery/healthy patient (Not life-threatening but potential for future morbidity and mortality. Requires in-hospital stay)	Postpone surgery if possible or consider ASC
	Tier 2b	Intermediate acuity surgery/unhealthy patient	Postpone surgery if possible or consider ASC
	Tier 3a	High acuity surgery/healthy patient	Do not postpone
	Tier 3b	High acuity surgery/unhealthy patient	Do not postpone

OPERATION THEATER

The risk to personnel is increased because of airborne spread. The recommendation for minimum personnel at time of induction is still applicable; it is logical even if there is no concrete data available in its favor. OT ventilation is achieved by increasing the number of air exchanges and HEPA filtration. OTs have been traditionally designed to have positive pressure air circulation, but there has been a trend towards negative pressure operating rooms since these would theoretically reduce the chances of spread of the virus to other operation theaters. The benefit of this step is yet to be proven, and nearly all OTs currently in use are of positive pressure type to avoid wound infections. In emergency setting when the patient has not been tested by RT-PCR, a negative pressure OT is still recommended.

In well maintained OTs 15–20 air changes per hour take place, which corresponds to 14–18 min wait to ensure clean operating theater air for the next patient and OT staff. At 10 air changes per minute, it needs about 30 min to reduce 99% air contamination.

Laminar flow/air conditioners in the OT should be started after induction of anesthesia and laminar airflow/air conditioners should be stopped 20 minutes before extubation. All airway devices should be removed in the operating theater and not in the recovery area.

Last year there was no clarity regarding spread of virus through bodily fluids. RT-PCR samples have been reported from bodily fluids, but to date infectivity has not been proven. It is safe to say that standard precautions (N95 mask and OT gowns) give adequate protection, and special equipment is not required. Cleaning with 1% sodium hypochlorite solution is recommended for OT tables and trolleys as soon as the patient is shifted.

A recent Expert panel Consensus from Association of Minimal Access Surgical Oncologists (AMASO) suggests Rule of 20, which is:
- 20 air changes per hour minimum (ideally >25) in the theater
- 20 minutes before intubation and extubation to keep AC and positive pressure switched off
- 20 minutes after intubation to enter OT for surgeons and nurses
- 20°C AC temperature setting
- 20 minutes minimum waiting time after patient is shifted out to start cleaning the theater

POSTOPERATIVE WARDS

The biggest challenge is to ensure adequate spacing between patients in wards. This can lead to refusal to admit some patients which are not deemed urgent. Patients should have minimum stay in wards; admit day before surgery, and discharge as early as possible. Undergraduate and postgraduate teaching will be an unfortunate casualty of this policy.

TIMING OF ELECTIVE SURGERY

Patients with perioperative SARS-CoV-2 infection are at increased risk of death and pulmonary complications following surgery. As the cumulative number of people who have had SARS-CoV-2 infection rises, it will be increasingly common for patients needing surgery to have previously had SARS-CoV-2 infection. In a large international global study comprising of 140,231 patients across 1674 hospitals in 116 countries, it was found that patients operated within 6 weeks of SARS-CoV-2 diagnosis were at an increased risk of 30-day postoperative mortality and 30-day postoperative pulmonary complications.

The time from SARS-CoV-2 diagnosis to surgery was 0–2 weeks in 1138 patients (36.4%), 3–4 weeks in 461 patients (14.7%), 5–6 weeks in 326 patients (10.4%) and ≥7 weeks in 1202 patients (38.4%). These risks decreased to baseline in patients who underwent surgery ≥7 weeks after SARS-CoV-2 diagnosis. These findings were consistent across both low-risk (age <70 years, ASA physical status 1–2, minor surgery) and high-risk (age ≥70 years, ASA physical status 3–5, major surgery) sub-groups.

Therefore, surgery should be delayed for at least 7 weeks following SARS-CoV-2 infection to reduce the risk of postoperative mortality and pulmonary complications. It was also found that patients who are still symptomatic ≥7 weeks after SARS-CoV-2 infection and undergo surgery also have an increased mortality rate. This study's findings support informed shared decision-making by anesthetists, surgeons and patients. Decisions should be tailored for each patient, since the possible advantages of delaying surgery for at least 7 weeks following SARS-CoV-2 diagnosis must be balanced against the potential risks of delay.

Research from a COVID surg prospective observational cohort study suggests that elective patients who develop hospital-acquired COVID-19 have a postoperative 30-day mortality of 16.2% with the two-thirds who experience pulmonary complications having a mortality rate of 23.8%. The rapid spread of COVID-19 around the world means that the notion of materiality must include a series of additional considerations which should be discussed with the patient as part of the informed consent process. These include:

a. The risk of contracting COVID-19 while in the hospital.
b. The risk of operation for patients who have tested positive for COVID-19.
c. Changes in the coordination of care due to the pandemic response and possible scarcity of resources (e.g. ICU bed capacity or ventilator availability).
d. The importance of advance directives.

The timing of elective surgery after recovery from COVID-19 utilizes both symptom- and severity-based categories. Suggested wait times from the date of COVID-19 diagnosis to surgery are as follows:

a. Four weeks for an asymptomatic patient or recovery from only mild, non-respiratory symptoms.
b. Six weeks for a symptomatic patient (e.g. cough, dyspnea) who did not require hospitalization.
c. Eight to ten weeks for a symptomatic patient who is diabetic, immunocompromised, or hospitalized.
d. Twelve weeks for a patient who was admitted to an intensive care unit due to COVID-19 infection.

These timelines should not be considered definitive; each patient's preoperative risk assessment should be individualized, factoring in surgical intensity, patient co-morbidities, and the benefit/risk ratio of further delaying surgery. Residual symptoms such as fatigue, shortness of breath, and chest pain are common in patients who have had COVID-19. These symptoms can be present more than 60 days after diagnosis, therefore patients with long covid should be assessed for cardiopulmonary function and surgical need be considered accordingly.

VACCINATION

Preoperative SARS-CoV-2 vaccination could support safer elective surgery. Vaccine numbers were limited initially so modelling techniques were used to assess priority. The primary outcome was the number needed to vaccinate (NNV) to prevent one COVID-19-related death in 1 year. NNVs were based on postoperative SARS-CoV-2 rates and mortality in an international cohort study (surgical patients), and community SARS-CoV-2 incidence and case fatality data (general population). NNV estimates were stratified by age (18–49, 50–69, 70 or more years) and type of surgery. Best- and worst-case scenarios were used to describe uncertainty.

NNV to prevent one COVID-19-related death over 30 days: Across age groups, NNVs were lowest in people aged 70 years or more: 425 (231 for best-case, 1080 for worst-case scenario) for those needing cancer surgery, 1157 (592, 3316) for those needing non-cancer surgery, and 22 384 (14 552, 37 302) for the general population.

NNV to prevent one COVID-19-related death over 1 year: NNVs to prevent one COVID-19-related death over 1 year were lower for surgical patients than the general population in all age groups. NNVs were lowest in people aged at least 70 years: 351 (196 for best-case, 816 for worst-case scenario) among those needing cancer surgery, 733 (407, 1664) for those needing non-cancer surgery, and 1840 (1196, 3066) for the general population. However, NNVs in patients aged 50–69 years needing either cancer surgery (559; 304, 1482) or non-cancer surgery (1621; 854, 4577) were favorable compared with the NNV for the general population aged 70 years or more.

There is no data to suggest superiority of one vaccine over the other with respect to postoperative outcomes. However, due to mutations it is desirable even fully vaccinated persons be tested before surgery, especially if there is a rising trend of cases in the city.

Currently, there are no national guidelines which require vaccination before surgery, simply because it is not possible to vaccinate the entire population quickly. It should be remembered that the primary role of vaccination is to reduce severity of disease; it does not prevent transmission. Hence, fully vaccinated persons may also spread disease. It is only when a significant percentage of population (>70% by some estimates) is vaccinated that a benefit is felt in society. Once vaccination targets are met, it is possible vaccinated persons will be given priority for elective surgery.

OPEN AND LAPAROSCOPIC SURGERY

Surgical smoke is widely known to harbor particulates of blood, bacteria, and viruses, and of numerous chemicals, such as benzene, formaldehyde, acrolein, and CO, among others apart from carcinogenic and neurotoxic compounds. Several reports have documented human papillomavirus (HPV) transmission to gynecologists or operating room nurse after laser ablation, and the presence of the hepatitis B virus (HBV) and human immunodeficiency virus have been confirmed in surgical smoke. Regrettably, most medical staff are not aware of the risks. Even though SARS-CoV-2 virus has never been found in surgical smoke, the risk of viral transmission cannot be excluded.

Surgical smoke, sometimes also referred to as plume, aerosol or vapor, is a surgically generated by-product of tissue combustion. The quantity of generated surgical smoke varies depending on the procedure being performed, the nature of the tissue and the surgical tool being used. The size of surgical smoke particles varies from 0.07 to 6.5 μm, depending on the device. It has been reported that small particles (0.07 μm) are produced by electrocautery, while large particles (0.35–6 μm) are produced by an ultrasonic scalpel. According to the Aerosol Consensus Statement, particles that are 5 μm or larger in size reach the nasopharynx, those sized 2–5 μm can be delivered to the airway, and those smaller than 3 μm reach the pulmonary parenchyma. It has been found in a study that both PM 2.5 and large PM were significantly more abundant in open surgery than in laparoscopic surgery.

Several associations have provided recommendations for laparoscopic surgery, and these include maintaining lower pneumoperitoneum pressure, minimizing the use of energy devices, avoiding long dissecting times, frequent suction to avoid the accumulation of smoke, and safety evacuation before trocar removal or laparotomy. In laparoscopic surgery, attention to surgical smoke is important during the extracorporeal procedure performed through a small laparotomy incision. It appears that high levels of PM can be released even in laparoscopic surgery. Thus, surgeons and operating room personnel should attempt to minimize any risk of transmission through surgical smoke during both open and laparoscopic surgeries. There is no scientific evidence to date for the transmission of COVID-19 by laparoscopic surgery. Laparoscopy can be used with precautions because of its benefits compared to open surgery.

The use of smoke evacuators with ULPA filters (remove 99.99% of the particles that measure 0.12 μm or more in diameter) is recommended for both open and laparoscopic surgery. It is not a substitute for personal precautions.

Society of American GI Endosurgeons (SAGES) Recommendations

- Consent discussion with patients must cover the risk of COVID-19 exposure and the potential consequences.
- If readily available and practical, surgical patients should be tested preoperatively for COVID-19.
- If needed and possible, intubation and extubation should take place within a negative pressure room.
- Operating rooms for presumed, suspected or confirmed COVID-19 positive patients should be appropriately filtered and ventilated and if possible, should be different than rooms used for other emergent surgical patients. Negative pressure rooms should be considered, if available.
- Only those considered essential staff should be participating in the surgical case and unless there is an emergency, there should be no exchange of room staff.
- All members of the OR staff should use PPE as recommended by national or international organization including the WHO or CDC. Appropriate gowns and face shields should be utilized. These measures should be used in all surgical procedures during the pandemic regardless of known or suspected COVID status. Placement and removal of PPE in should be done according to CDC guidelines.

- Electrosurgery units should be set to the lowest possible settings for the desired effect. Use of monopolar electrosurgery, ultrasonic dissectors, and advanced bipolar devices should be minimized, as these can lead to particle aerosolization. If available, monopolar diathermy pencils with attached smoke evacuators should be used.
- Surgical equipment used during procedures with COVID-19 positive or persons under investigation (PUI)/suspected COVID patients should be cleaned separately from other surgical equipment.

PRACTICAL MEASURES FOR LAPAROSCOPY

- Incisions for ports should be as small as possible to allow for the passage of ports but not allow for leakage around ports.
- CO_2 insufflation pressure should be kept to a minimum and an ultrafiltration (smoke evacuation system or filtration) should be used, if available.
- All pneumoperitoneum should be safely evacuated via a filtration system before closure, trocar removal, specimen extraction or conversion to open.

CHECKLIST

The surgical safety checklist (most commonly WHO checklist) is used in many healthcare facilities; the current pandemic has forced are think beyond the routine checklist and a modified surgical safety checklist has been developed by lifebox, the World Federation of Societies of Anaesthesiogists, and Smile Train. It has pertinent points related to operation on COVID patients (Addendum).

CONCLUSION

COVID-19 has changed the way we practise surgery, and the changes are likely to remain in force for coming many years. Personal protection and measures to prevent cross infection should become part and parcel of a surgeon's life. It is also the duty of every medical professional to promote good practices in everyday living.

New evidence is continuously emerging and guidelines are being modified and updated regularly. The readers are therefore urged to refer to the most recent versions of the guidelines and resources as the evidence evolves.

SUGGESTING READING

1. Air changes/hour (ACH) and time required for airborne-contaminant removal by efficiency.https://www.cdc.gov/infectioncontrol/guidelines/environmental/appendix/air.html
2. Antunes D, Lami M, Chukwudi A, Dey A, Patel M, Shabana A, Shams M, Slack Z, Bond-Smith G, Tebala G. COVID-19 infection risk by open and laparoscopic surgical smoke: A systematic review of the literature. Surgeon. 2021 Mar 3:S1479-666X(21)00041-X. doi: 10.1016/j.surge.2021.02.003. Epub ahead of print.
3. ASA and APSF Joint Statement on Elective Surgery and Anesthesia for Patients after COVID-19 Infection available from https://www.asahq.org/about-asa/newsroom/news-releases/2020/12/asa-and-apsf-joint-statement-on-elective-surgery-and-anesthesia-for-patients-after-COVID-19-infection
4. ASI's Consensus Guidance document. ABCs of what to do and what not during the COVID-19 pandemic.

5. Bains L, Mishra A, Gupta L, Singh R, Lal P. Surgery in COVID 19 Times: A Comprehensive Review. MAMC J MedSci 2020;6:163–75.

6. COVID-19 Surgical Patient Checklist. Accessed from https://www.lifebox.org/covid/covid-19-surgical-patient-checklist/

7. COVID-19: Guidance for Triage of Non-Emergent Surgical Procedures. Accessed from https://www.facs.org/covid-19/clinical-guidance/triage on 17 July 2020.

8. El Boghdady M, Ewalds-Kvist BM. Laparoscopic surgery and the debate on its safety during COVID-19 pandemic: A systematic review of recommendations. Surgeon. 2021 Apr;19(2):e29-e39. doi: 10.1016/j.surge.2020.07.005.

9. Francis, N Dort J, Cho E, et al. SAGES and EAES recommendations for minimally invasive surgery during COVID 19 pandemic. Surg Endosc 34, 2327–2331 (2020). https://doi.org/10.1007/s00464-020-07565-w

10. Greenhalgh T, Jimenez JL, Prather KA, Tufekci Z, Fisman D, Schooley R. Ten scientific reasons in support of airborne transmission of SARS-CoV-2. Lancet. 2021 May 1;397(10285):1603–5. doi: 10.1016/S0140-6736(21)00869-2. Epub 2021 Apr 15. Erratum in: Lancet. 2021 May 15;397(10287):1808. PMID: 33865497; PMCID: PMC8049599

11. Intercollegiate General Surgery Guidance on COVID-19. Accessed from https://www.rcseng.ac.uk/coronavirus/joint-guidance-for-surgeons-v2/ on 20 May 2020.

12. Kameyama H, Otani T, Yamazaki T, et al. Comparison of surgical smoke between open surgery and laparoscopic surgery for colorectal disease in the COVID-19 era. Surg Endosc (2021). https://doi.org/10.1007/s00464-021-08394-1.

13. Moletta L, Pierobon ES, Capovilla G, et al. International guidelines and recommendations for surgery during COVID-19 pandemic: A Systematic Review. Int J Surg. 2020;79:180–8. doi:10.1016/j.ijsu.2020.05.061

14. NHS. 2020. Clinical Guide to Surgical Prioritization during the Coronavirus Pandemic.https://www.england.nhs.uk/coronavirus/wp-content/uploads/sites/52/2020/03/C0221-specialty-guide-surgical-prioritisation-v1.pdf accessed 25 April 2020.

15. SAGES Practical Measures for Surgery available at https://www.sages.org/recommendations-surgical-response-covid-19/

16. SARS-CoV-2 vaccination modelling for safe surgery to save lives: data from an international prospective cohort study. Br J Surg. 2021 Mar 24;znab101. doi: 10.1093/bjs/znab101. Online ahead of print.

17. Srivastava A, Nasta AM, Pathania BS, Sundaram E, Jani KV, Manickavasagam K, Asuri K, Lal P, Goel RG, Chaudhari T, Bansal VK. Surgical practice recommendations for minimal access surgeons during COVID-19 pandemic–Indian inter-society directives. J Min Access Surg2020;16:195–200.

18. Timing of surgery following SARS-CoV-2 infection: an international prospective cohort study. Anaesthesia. 2021 Jun;76(6):748–58. doi: 10.1111/anae.15458.

Renal Involvement in COVID-19

Himansu Sekhar Mahapatra, Renju Binoy

INTRODUCTION

Coronavirus disease 2019 (COVID-19) is an acute respiratory infection caused by a novel betacoronavirus named SARS-CoV-2 (severe acute respiratory syndrome coronavirus 2), which is thought to be originated at the seafood market in Wuhan, Hubei Province of China. It has been estimated that, as of August 11, 2020, more than 20 million (20,254,662) individuals have been infected and is responsible for 7,38,930 casualties worldwide. Among six coronavirus species, which are known to cause human disease, four viruses (229E, OC43, NL63 and HKU1) typically cause common cold symptoms in immunocompetent individuals, other two strains are SARS-CoV and Middle East respiratory syndrome coronavirus (MERS-CoV) which are zoonotic in origin and have been linked to sometimes fatal illness. The new virus causing COVID-19 has been found to be genetically and phylogenetically similar, but not identical, to the SARS-CoV causing SARS disease and hence was named SARS-CoV-2 by the International Committee on Taxonomy of Viruses (ICTV). SARS-CoV-2 is primarily spread from person to person through respiratory droplets, which are typically released when an infected person coughs or sneezes. Transmission may also occur through fomites in the immediate environment around the infected person. According to the World Health Organization (WHO), the incubation period for COVID-19, is on an average 5–6 days, however, can be up to 14 days.

In 30th January 2020, the first case of COVID-19, a student returning from Wuhan, China, was reported in India. By 11th August, there are now more than 2 million cases and 45,353 casualties, with Maharashtra, Tamil Nadu and Andhra Pradesh being the worst affected with an upward slope in morbidity and mortality. India with its 1.3 billion population, and a high prevalence of comorbidities like diabetes, hypertension and chronic kidney disease (CKD), can become the new epicenter of the virus. According to the data from the International Society of Nephrology's Kidney Disease Data Center Study, the reported prevalence of CKD in India is 17% and that of end-stage renal disease (ESRD) is 2.9%, in whom COVID-19 can be deadly. Even though COVID-19 is a systemic disease, lungs and kidneys seem to be the organs most to bear the blunt.

PATHOGENESIS OF RENAL INVOLVEMENT IN COVID-19

SARS-CoV-2 enters human cells through the angiotensin-converting–enzyme 2 (ACE2) receptor. S-protein of SARS-CoV-2 binds to host cell receptors ACE2, which is a critical step for virus entry. After membrane fusion, the viral genome RNA is released into the cytoplasm, and the uncoated RNA translates two polyproteins, pp1a and pp1ab, which encode nonstructural proteins, and form replication-transcription complex (RTC) in double-membrane vesicle. Continuously RTC replicates and synthesizes a nested set of subgenomic RNAs, which encode accessory proteins and structural proteins. With the help of endoplasmic reticulum (ER) and Golgi bodies, newly formed genomic RNA, nucleocapsid proteins, and envelope glycoproteins assemble and form viral particle buds. Lastly, the virion-containing vesicles fuse with the plasma membrane to release the virus leading to viremia.

The mechanism of kidney injury by COVID-19 appears multifactorial and, although precisely, remains unknown. The direct viral cytopathic effect on kidney tissue is a postulated mechanism, which is supported by the finding of viral particles in tubular epithelial cells and podocytes by EM in autopsied patients who have died of COVID-19. It is a fact that ACE2 expression is 100-fold higher in kidney tissues than the lung. The other major mechanism of action could be by inducing sepsis and the resultant cytokine storm. The cytokines and other mediators released after SARS-CoV-2 infection may lead to sustained inflammatory response, which in turn can culminate in shock, hypoxia, rhabdomyolysis and multiple organ dysfunction. Another postulated hypothesis is the direct effector T cell-mediated injury and the immune complex-mediated glomerular injury with viral antigen and specific antibody. However, the present evidence of information with normal glomeruli on autopsies and absence of electron-dense deposit in SARS-CoV-2 patients, do not support this hypothesis.

The effect of COVID-19 on kidney can be categorized into three main headings:
1. Acute kidney disease (AKI) in patients with COVID-19.
2. CKD patients and those patients on maintenance hemodialysis getting infected with COVID-19.
3. Renal transplant patients getting infected with COVID-19.

AKI in Patients with COVID-19

According to the latest estimates, 80% of people with COVID-19 will have mild or moderate disease (including people without pneumonia and people with mild pneumonia), 15% will have severe disease and 5% will have critical illness. Even though SARS-CoV-2 mainly affects the respiratory tract, it can affect multiple organs either directly or indirectly. SARS-CoV-2 can affect the kidneys either directly (as ACE-2 receptors are also present in kidney) or indirectly (as part of cytokine storm).

In an earlier report, of 138 patients with COVID-19, a total of 5 patients (3.6%) had AKI. Out of 36 patients requiring ICU care, 3 (8.3%) had AKI. In another study by Cheng et al of 701 patients who were observed prospectively. One percent patients developed AKI, 43.9% of patients had proteinuria and 26.7% had hematuria at the time of admission. The prevalence of elevated serum creatinine, elevated blood urea nitrogen and estimated glomerular filtration under 60 ml/min/1.73 m² at the time of admission were 14.4%, 13.1% and 13.1%, respectively. Patients with proteinuria and hematuria were 43.9% and 26.7%. Sixty-three percent of patients with AKI develop proteinuria, of which 34% is nephrotic range. When adjusted for age, sex, comorbidity, leukocyte count and disease severity, presence of AKI, proteinuria and hematuria were independent risk factors for in-hospital death. The risk of mortality as expectedly increased with the stage of AKI.

An autopsy study of 26 COVID-19 patients who expired of respiratory failure by Su et al, approximately one-third of patients (9/26) had kidney dysfunction prior to death. Only 9 of the patients had a premorbid urinalysis. Seven of 9 had proteinuria and 6 of 9 had hematuria. All cases in the series showed mild-to-severe acute tubular injury. Acute tubular injury was characterized by a loss of the proximal tubular brush borders, vacuolar degeneration (non-isometric in most cases), coagulative necrosis (4 cases), hemosiderin granules within tubular cytoplasm and pigmented casts within tubular lumens. Two cases showed evidence of acute pyelonephritis, with neutrophil-rich interstitial inflammation, bacterial colonies within kidney parenchyma and abscess formation. There was evidence of glomerular ischemia, with three of the cases show fibrin thrombi within the glomerular capillary loops. No proliferative changes were identified within glomeruli, such as endocapillary hypercellularity or true crescents (cellular or fibrocellular). Ultrastructural analysis by electron microscopy revealed presence of virions in the podocytes and tubular epithelial cells, consistent with direct infection of kidney parenchyma and subendothelial electron-lucent widening suggestive of endothelial injury. Virions were characterized by being 65–136 nm in size, with 20–25 nm spikes and a solar 'corona' configuration.

The indication for renal replacement therapy (RRT) is not much different from other causes of AKI. As per the Guidelines issued by the COVID-19 Working Group of Indian Society of Nephrology, all modalities of RRT may be used for patients with AKI depending on their clinical status. Patients admitted in other wards of the hospital with AKI should be preferably given bedside dialysis rather than shifting patient in main dialysis unit. In such situation portable reverse osmosis water in a tank will serve the purpose for the dialysis. If more dialysis are expected in selected area, dialysis machine may be left in the same area for future use. Use of acute peritoneal dialysis can be life saving and should be used as and when required and, in the setting, where hemodialysis facility is not available. Healthcare worker should use all precaution while initiating acute peritoneal dialysis and discard used consumable properly. It has been observed that patients with COVID-19 are having a pro-coagulant state and hence the concern of clotting of the filter should be always kept in mind.

CKD Patients and Patients on Maintenance Hemodialysis with COVID-19

COVID-19 infection in patients with pre-existing disease like CKD is more severe than those patients without any comorbidities. This may be due to the attenuated immunity in these patients, poor nutritional status or the drugs these patients are on, some of which are immunosuppressants.

CKD was observed in 3% at admission in a cohort study with 1,591 patients (median age 63 years) with laboratory-confirmed COVID-19 admitted to ICU in Lombardy, Italy, between February 20 and March 18, 2020. CKD was reported in 4.7% and ESRD in 3.2% at admission in 5,700 patients (median age 63 years, 60.3% males) with confirmed COVID-19 admitted to 12 hospitals in New York City between March 1 and April 4, 2020. A meta-analysis conducted by Henry et al of 1,389 COVID-19 patients, presence of CKD was associated with an odds ratio of 3.03 for having severe disease.

Many patients of CKD will experience episodes of AKI after COVID-19 infection, and the renal function will deteriorate after infection leading to acute on CKD. Such a decline in kidney function depends on the severity of the infection.

One of the important considerations in these patients is whether to continue on renin-angiotensin-aldosterone system (RAAS) blocker or not, as the ACE-2 seems to be the receptor through which the virus gains entry into the cells. Most of these patients would be on RAAS blockers, as they are considered first-choice drugs in hypertension, heart failure, postmyocardial infarction states and CKD. But its known that ACE inhibitors or angiotensin receptor blockers (ARBs) increase the expression of ACE-2 on the membrane surface. But as of the evidence right now, its use has not been associated with increased incidence of the disease, severity or mortality. A population-based case-control study by Mancia et al in Italy, investigated for any correlation of RAAS blocker with COVID-19. They found, the use of ACE inhibitors and ARBs was more common among case patients than among controls, as was the use of other antihypertensive and nonantihypertensive drugs, indicating the correlation of comorbidities with COVID-19. There was also no relationship between ARB or ACE inhibitor use and severity of disease or mortality. So as of now, all the guidelines recommend continuing RAAS blockers unless contraindicated for other reasons.

In patients undergoing maintenance hemodialysis COVID-19 can be particularly lethal. Using data retrospectively collected from a registration system that included 7,154 patients undergoing hemodialysis at 65 hospitals in Wuhan, China, a study by Xiong et al found that 154 patients had laboratory-confirmed COVID-19. In a detailed analysis of epidemiologic and clinical characteristics for 131 COVID-19 patients who provided oral consent, they showed that hemodialysis centers are high-risk settings for COVID-19. They also observed that 13.8% of patients developed ARDS, which is higher than the rate for general population.

Management of patients on dialysis should be carried by strict adherence to guidelines issued by the COVID-19 Working Group of Indian Society of Nephrology, to minimize spread of infection. Patients on maintenance hemodialysis should be advised to adhere to their regular schedule to avoid any emergency dialysis. Patients should be informed about the symptoms of COVID-19 and should be encouraged to report to their unit before arriving via a phone. Stable patients on maintenance hemodialysis should be advised to come to the unit alone without any attendant. Every hemodialysis unit should contain a designated screening area, where the patients are questioned regarding any symptoms related to COVID-19 or any contact with COVID-19.

Patients with low suspicion for COVID-19

All patients should be advised to wear a three-layered surgical mask. Before dialysis, patients should wash their hands with soap and water for at least 20 seconds, using proper method of handwashing. If soap and water are not readily available, a hand sanitizer containing at least 60% alcohol can be used. Patients should follow cough etiquettes, like coughing or sneezing using the inside of the elbow or using tissue paper. Adequate spacing between the patients should be maintained. The staff caring for these patients should also be wearing a three-layered surgical mask. They should also wash their hands or use alcohol-based hand sanitizer in between 2 patients. Stethoscope diaphragms and tubing may be cleaned with an alcohol-based disinfectant including hand rubs in between patients. The bedlinen should be changed between shifts and used linen and gowns be placed in a dedicated container for waste or linen before leaving the dialysis station. Disposable gowns should be discarded after use. Cloth gowns should be soaked in a 1% hypochlorite solution for 20 minutes before sluicing and then be transported for laundering after each use. The guidelines recommend cleaning and disinfecting, the frequently touched surfaces at least thrice daily and after every shift. The solutions for disinfection be composed either of hypochlorite, alcohol, formaldehyde or glutaraldehyde for disinfection of surfaces in accordance with the manufacturer's instructions.

Patients who are suspected to be having COVID-19

Those patients, who are suspected to be having COVID-19 based on the screening, should be advised to undergo testing for COVID-19. They should undergo dialysis in isolation. The isolation ideally should be in a separate room with a closed door but may not be possible in all units. The next most suitable option is the use of a separate shift, preferably the last of the day for dialyzing all such patients. Where this is also not possible, suspected patient may be dialyzed at a row end within the unit ensuring a separation from all other patients by at least 2 meters. The patient should be wearing a mask preferably a N95 mask. The staff caring for these patients should be wearing the full PPE and preferably a N95 mask and should not care for other patients. If N95 masks are in short supply, they can be prioritized for use during aerosol generating procedures like intubation or nebulization. The instruments used for these patients should not also be used for other patients. If the test report of the patient comes as negative, they should be shifted to the regular dialysis area. In case of healthcare worker accidentally came in contact with a COVID-19 patient, he/she should be advised for testing as per the guidelines and should be put in quarantine pending arrival of the report.

Patients who are COVID-19 positive

Dialysis of patients with COVID-19 are advised to be done at the bedside, rather than at the unit, as mentioned earlier. If that is not possible should be done in isolation. But as the number of cases goes on increasing and without any signs of abating, a separate shift or even better a separate unit may be needed. Staff who is managing COVID-19 patients should be fully equipped with PPE, shoe covers, goggles or face shields and preferably a N95 mask.

COVID-19 and Renal Transplant Recipients

Kidney-transplant recipients appear to be at particularly high-risk for critical COVID-19 illness due to chronic immunosuppression and coexisting conditions. In a report by Akalin et al, of a total of 36 renal transplant recipients with COVID-19, 8 patients were in stable condition without major respiratory symptoms (22%) and were monitored at home and 28 patients (78%) were admitted to the hospital. Eleven (39%) of the hospitalized patients received mechanical ventilation. Six patients (21%) received RRT. At a median follow-up of 21 days (range, 14–28), 10 of those 36 kidney-transplant recipients (28%) and 7 of the 11 patients who were intubated (64%) had died.

For renal transplant recipients hospitalized with COVID-19 pneumonitis, the best practice would be that proposed by the Brescia Renal COVID Task Force, which includes withdrawal of antimetabolite-mycophenolate mofetil (MMF) or azathioprine (AZA) and calcineurin inhibitors and mammalian target of rapamycin (mTOR) inhibitors and continue replacement therapy with methylprednisolone 16 mg daily.

CONCLUSION

COVID-19 is a communicable respiratory disease caused by the virus SARS-CoV-2. Earlier reports are indicating about 5% incidence of AKI and is a strong and independent predictor of mortality. The pathogenesis of renal involvement is thought to be due to direct viral cytopathic effects and those due to cytokine storm. The dialysis for COVID-19 suspected and positive patients should be done according to the guidelines published by Indian Society of Nephrology. Transplant patients unfortunately are at greater risk for having a severe illness and may be managed with temporary cessation of immunosuppression. The greater challenge would be in providing RRT in positive or suspected patients as the cases are rising and may require innovative ideas like isolation dialysis units or dedicated days in existing units for positive patients.

Pregnancy and COVID-19 Infection

Niharika Dhiman, Krishna Agarwal, Chetna A Sethi, Asmita M Rathore

In these unprecedented times of COVID pandemic, health system around the world are overstretched. Health services for women and children are among the first to be affected. Early available data did not indicate that pregnant individuals were at an increased risk of infection or severe morbidity compared with non-pregnant individuals in the general population. However latest data from two studies by Hantoushzadeh *et al* (Case Series) and Elshafeey *et al* (Systematic Review) highlighted that most patients may have mild illness, but few of them may require intensive care.

EFFECT OF PREGNANCY ON COVID INFECTION

The clinical course of COVID -19 during pregnancy is unpredictable and may progress very fast in cases associated with medical comorbidities. The following anatomical and physiological changes during pregnancy may predispose a pregnant woman to the infection.

i. Under the effect of progesterone and other relaxants in pregnancy causes relaxation of the ligaments of the ribs, with the progressive increases in size of uterus the diaphragm is pushed up and the transverse diameter of the chest increases which leads to eventually lead to a 20 to 30% reduction in functional residual capacity (FRC), which makes the mother prone to hypoxia, subsequently compensated by increased tidal volume and hyperventilation.

ii. It has been postulated that in the later half of pregnancy is characterized by a decreased number and activity in NK cells and T cells, which may affect the viral clearance rate and lays a foundation for the onset and deterioration of infectious diseases in later half of the pregnancy as seen in the previous pandemics of SARS-CoVi-1 and H1N1.

iii. It is speculated that level of ACE2 is doubled during pregnancy to regulate blood pressure. This adaptation may be a favorable condition for SARS-CoV-2 infection. ACE2 is not only a receptor, but also involved in postinfection regulation, including immune response, cytokine secretion, and viral genome replication.

EFFECT OF COVID INFECTION ON PREGNANCY

i. Maternal: There are increased chances of cesarean section, FGR (fetal growth restriction), preterm labor and fetal distress however the evidence is still limited.

ii. Fetal: The chances of vertical transmission is still not established.

iii. Care of COVID positive pregnant woman.

At the point of admission confirmed cases need to be assessed and risk stratification to be done depending upon the clinical presentation and triage to be done according to the National Early Warning Score (NEWS) 2.

Every confirmed case of COVID-19 (MoHFW) should be manged according to the following principles (Table 12.1).

TABLE 12.1: Principle of management of COVID positive pregnant woman

Clinical syndrome	Definition	Management principles
Mild illness	Uncomplicated upper respiratory tract viral infection may have non-specific symptoms—fever, cough, sore throat, nasal congestion, headache, or malaise **NO breathlessness**	a. Adequate nutrition and hydration b. Symptomatic management like antipyretics and antihistaminic c. Tab Hydroxychloroquine (HCQ) may be considered for women having high-risk factors (hypertension, diabetes, chronic lung/kidney/ liver disease, cerebrovascular disease or obesity under strict medical supervision d. If worsening symptoms, urgent medical care should be given
Moderate illness	Pneumonia with no signs of severe disease. Presence of breathlessness and or features of hypoxia (Respiratory Rate 24/minute, SpO_2 90%–96% on room air) 12-lead ECG- daily CBC, absolute lymphocyte count, KFT and LFT-daily CRP, D-dimer and Ferritin every 48–72 hours	a. Monitoring and supportive care to be provided b. Oxygen by nasal cannula or mask with breathing or non-rebreathing reservoir bag c. Maintenance IV fluids d. Awake proning till 20 weeks of pregnancy, semi-recumbent position with a slight left lateral tilt after 20 weeks of pregnancy e. Antibiotics to cover organisms known to cause community based pneumonia (cap Amoxiclav 625 mg TDS for 7 days) f. Azithromycin 500 mg OD for 5 days g. Tab Hydroxychloroquine 400 mg BD on day 1 followed by 200 mg BD for 4 days h. IV methylprednisolone 0.5–1 mg/kg /day for 3 days in consultation with medicine consultant i. Prophylactic anticoagulation in consultation with medicine consultant-enoxaparin 40 mg per day SC or unfractionated heparin 5000 IU SC 12 hourly
Severe illness	Severe pneumonia-breathlessness with respiratory rate ≥30/minute and/or SpO_2 <90% in room air	a. Admitted in COVID-19 ICU and receive treatment as per standard treatment protocol

(Contd.)

TABLE 12.1: Principle of management of COVID positive pregnant woman (Contd.)

Clinical syndrome	Definition	Management principles
		b. Oxygen therapy by nasal cannula or mask with breathing or non-rebreathing reservoir bag at rate of 5 L/min with target SpO_2 94% but not exceding 96% c. Antibiotics to cover organisms known to cause community based pneumonia IV ceftriaxone 2 gm IV BD d. Early short course of IV methylprednisolone 0.5–1 mg/kg /day for 3 days in consultation with treating physician[§] *Or* Tab Dexamethasone 6 mg PO once a day for 6–10 days[§] e. Prophylactic anticoagulation enoxaparin 40 mg per day SC or unfractionated heparin 5000 IU SC 12 hourly. Higher doses can be given in severe illness f. Specific therapy related to use of convalescent plasma, Remdesivir (a nucleotide analogue prodrug that inhibits viral RNA polymerases) should be considered in consultation with physician[§]
	Hypoxemic respiratory failure and acute respiratory distress syndrome (ARDS)	i. Initiate high-flow nasal cannula oxygenation (HFNO) or noninvasive mechanical ventilation if not responding to standard oxygen therapy ii. If does not improve over then intubation and invasive ventilation should be performed
	Sepsis	Higher antibiotics for broad-spectrum coverage
	Septic Shock	a. Fluid therapy—RL or NS IV fluids –30 ml/kg over first 3 hours b. Prevent fluid overload—aiming daily negative balance of 0.5–1 L c. Vasopressor to be started if fluid therapy is not sufficient. Inotrope dopamine may be given if still poor perfusion persists

[§]Limited evidence available for use in pregnancy and postpartum period however have been used on compassionate grounds.

Antenatal corticosteroids can be given between 24 and 34 weeks in women at risk of preterm labor provided there is no risk of worsening of maternal condition. Tocolytics should be avoided. Treatment may be individualized according to the patient profile at the discretion of treating obstetrician.

INTRAPARTUM CARE FOR COVID POSITIVE WOMEN

i. Repeat risk stratification and assessment of severity of COVID 19 symptoms (Table 12.2).

ii. The mode and timing of delivery is individualized. Covid infection per se is not an indication for termination of pregnancy.

iii. Mother must wear surgical mask and be shifted to the designated delivery room.

TABLE 12.2: Intrapartum care according to severity of illness

	No/mild illness	Moderate/severe illness
Maternal monitoring		*Priority is to stabilize woman's condition with standard care therapy*
i. Temperature ii. Pulse rate iii. Respiratory rate iv. Blood pressure	—As per routine protocol—	Hourly monitoring
v. SpO$_2$ vi. ABG vii. I/O charting	SpO$_2$–Hourly (Aim: >94%) ABG–Baseline	Continuous SpO$_2$ monitoring (Aim: >94%) ABG baseline and repeat as required I/O charting: Hourly, avoid fluid overload Preanesthetic check up to be done
Investigations	i. As per routine protocol for laboring women ii. Sepsis screen as per clinical indication iii. PT, aPTT, CRP, D-dimer and ferritin every 48–72 hours, IL-6, Pro-calcitonin (prediction of cytokiene storm) iv. Chest X-ray and CT of chest with abdominal shield, if indicated in moderate to severe cases	
Mode of delivery	Cesarean section only for obstetric indication. Regional anesthesia is preferred.	In case cesarean section is **indicated**: i. To assist efforts in maternal resuscitation ii. For serious concerns for fetal condition *Decision to be made by consultants of MDT considering the following:* a. Maternal condition b. Fetal viability c. Potential improvement following cesarean section **Priority must be the well-being of mother**
Antibiotic prophylaxis	Other than specific COVID therapy and antibiotics for coverage for community based pneumonia, drugs to be individualized in consultation with physician.	
Induction of labor	—As per routine protocol—	
Labor monitoring	—As per routine protocol—	
Fetal monitoring-hand held Doppler/CTG	—As per routine protocol—	
Second stage of labor	Cut short second stage of labor if woman is symptomatic (exhausted/hypoxic)	
Third stage of labor	AMTL and delayed cord clamping	

iv. Women admitted in ICU need to be delivered in ICU under close supervision of the obstetric team.

v. All healthcare workers must wear full PPE (N95 mask, shoe covers, goggles, gown and head gear).

vi. The members of multidisciplinary team (obstetrician, physician, anesthetist and neonatologist) are to be informed.

vii. PPH management tools: Uterotonics (Tab. Misoprostol, Inj. Syntocinon, Inj. Ergometrine), Balloon tamponade kit and cervical exploration tray to be kept ready during delivery.

viii. Number of staff entering the designated delivery area should be kept to minimum and all should wear PPE.

CESAREAN SECTION FOR COVID POSITIVE WOMEN

1. Number of staff in the operation area to be kept to minimum, all of whom should wear appropriate PPE.
2. All team members should have been trained prior in donning and doffing PPE.
3. Team members: Obstetrician–2, Neonatologist–1, Anesthetist–2, OT staff: Technician–1, Scrub Nurse–1, Circulating Staff–1.
4. Each team member to be labelled with designation/name as verbal communication after donning PPE is difficult.
5. Sequence of entering OT: Scrub nurse and OT technician to enter first to prepare trolley and other requirements.
6. Neonatologist to ensure neonatal resuscitation kit. Only anesthesia team to be present in the OT during administration of anesthesia. Followed by the obstetricians.
7. Appropriate disposal of PPE to be done.

POSTPARTUM CARE FOR COVID POSITIVE WOMEN

a. Neonatal resuscitation corner should be located at least **2 m** away from the delivery table.
b. Mother should perform hand hygiene and wear triple layer mask, practice respiratory hygiene and the surfaces should be periodically cleaned.
c. Healthy neonate may be roomed-in with mother who has no or mild symptoms.
d. Direct breastfeeding can be given. Mother should wash hands frequently including before breastfeeding and should wear surgical mask.

However the couple should be given the option of deciding whether the baby should be roomed in with the mother or given to a healthy relative.

DISCHARGE POLICY

a. Women who had normal delivery can be discharged after 48 hours of birth and women who had cesarean delivery can be discharged after four days of cesarean section, whenever she is fit for discharge and need not to wait negative COVID-19 test.

b. Asymptomatic antenatal women who do not need hospital care can be discharged for home isolation (14 days) after fulfilling all the prerequisites (no symptom onset within next 10 days and no fever × 3 days) and should follow in COVID or Non-COVID hospital according to their subsequent test results.

c. Moderate disease: Can be discharged in absence of fever without antipyretics, resolution of breathlessness and no oxygen requirement.

d. Severe disease: Discharge will be based on-clinical recovery and patient tested negative once by RT-PCR (after resolution of symptoms).

RECORD KEEPING

A record of total admissions, number of deliveries, cesarean sections, stillbirths and maternal mortality should be maintained and timely audit done for the same.

MAMC Experience

Suresh Kumar, Anil Chokan, Rajesh Ruttala

At the time of writing, a total of 21,600 patients (COVID-19 suspected plus confirmed positive cases) have been admitted in LNJP Hospital, Delhi. As per the directions of Delhi Government, LNJP has been converted into a dedicated COVID-19 hospital, thereby recruiting manpower in the form of experienced faculty, residents, nursing staff and other healthcare workers in tackling this huge pandemic.

Total number of patients admitted in LNH is 21,600 out of these 20,500 patients successfully discharged.

The plan of action has been as follows:

- The main casualty is now serving as point of care for COVID-19 suspected patients where a team of doctors and nursing staff is deployed round the clock.
- From thereon, further segregation is done on the basis of disease severity and patients are shifted to different indoor facilities depending on red, orange and green categories.
- All red category (severe) patients are shifted to the ICU.
- Dedicated staff for COVID care has been arranged in ICU where a team of highly skillful anesthetists, intensivists and team of all specialists with specially trained nurses are available for round the clock duty with state-of-the-art facilities.

Number of patients admitted	21600
Number of patients successfully discharged	20500
Number of dialysis sessions	2151
Number of lower segment cesarean section	266
Number of nomal vaginal deliveries	361
Post COVID syndrome	219
Mucormycosis	240
Vaccination	35,800

Besides the standard medical treatment, we at MAMC have conducted trials on experimental therpaies like convalescent plasma (1 completed and 1 ongoing) and biologics like Itolizumab. As new drugs are getting approved in light of latest recommendation, Remdesivir and Tocilizumab have also been included in the treatment armamentorium agaisnt COVID-19.

CONVALESCENT PLASMA

Patients with moderate-to-severe disease were enrolled in this randomized controlled trial (RCT) after formal consent and careful scrutiny of inclusion and exclusion criterias. Convalescent plasma was procured in collaboration with Institute of Liver and Biliary Sciences (ILBS), New Delhi and the same was transfused to the patients in the treatment arm. Patients were then monitored for clinical improvement or deterioration. Laboratory parameters were also simultaneously studied in both the treatment as well as control arms.

Following is the flow diagram of the procedure followed in the aforementioned trial:

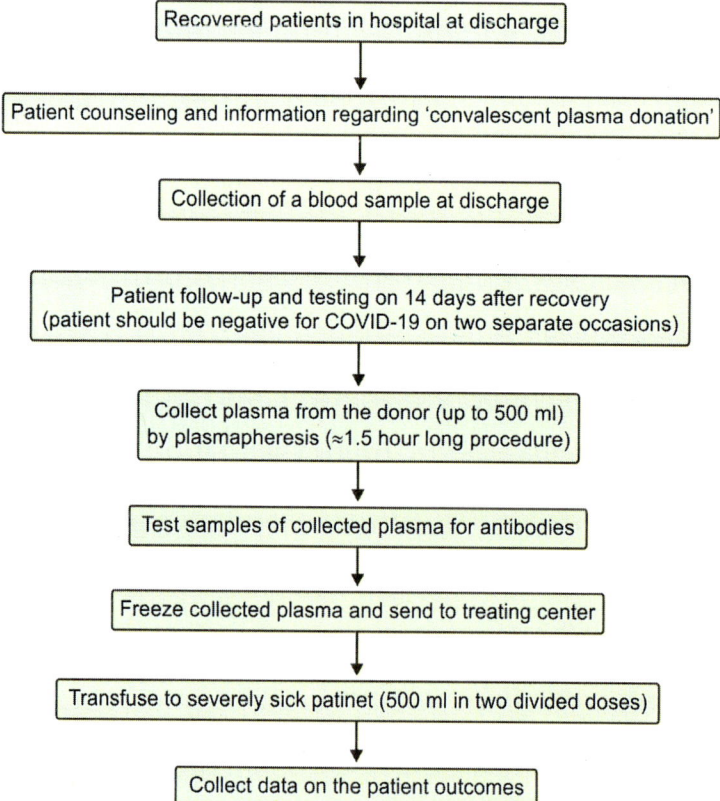

ITOLIZUMAB

Itolizumab is an anti-CD6 humanized IgG1 monoclonal antibody. Itolizumab has a potent anti-inflammatory effect reducing the production of pro-inflammatory cytokines interleukin (IL)-6, tumor necrosis factor (TNF), interferon (IFN)-γ, IL-17 and IL-1. Itolizumab in COVID-19 patients theoretically has the potential to control the pro-inflammatory cytokine storm syndrome, by immunomodulation of Teff function and trafficking to the inflammation site, sparing Tregs and preserving the antiviral response, reducing the morbidity and mortality. In the RCT conducted in our center, patients with moderate-to-severe ARDS were enrolled and were randomized to treatment and control (standard medical treatment) groups. Patients with active or latent tuberculosis, HIV/hepatitis B or hepatitis C infections were excluded from the study. Itolizumab in doses of 1.6 mg/kg as an IV infusion was administered to the subjects in the treatment arm. Subsequently, weekly doses of 0.8 mg/kg were given to patients till clinical improvement. One-month mortality was compared between the two groups. Biochemical parameters like IL-6, TNF-α, IL-1, IL-17 levels were also monitored in both the groups and compared.

The results of the above-mentioned studies are yet to be published although some initial promise has been shown. Significantly larger number of patients at multiple centers need to be studied in order to extrapolate the results to the wider population.

DIGITALIZATION AND MENTAL HEALTH INITIATIVE

In light of effects of the COVID-19 pandemic on the mental health of both patients as well as healthcare workers, it becomes the duty of policy makers and institution management to provide for optimal psychological counseling for anyone suffering from psychological distress directly or indirectly related to this pandemic. A Mental Health Initiative has been launched by MAMC-LNH to provide for psychological counseling for all residents working in COVID-19 wards.

Besides this, all the designated COVID wards have been provided with a Tablet phone for the purpose of video calling to ensure patients remain in touch with their families in these unprecedented times.

SECOND WAVE (ALL INDIA) COVID POSITIVE CASES

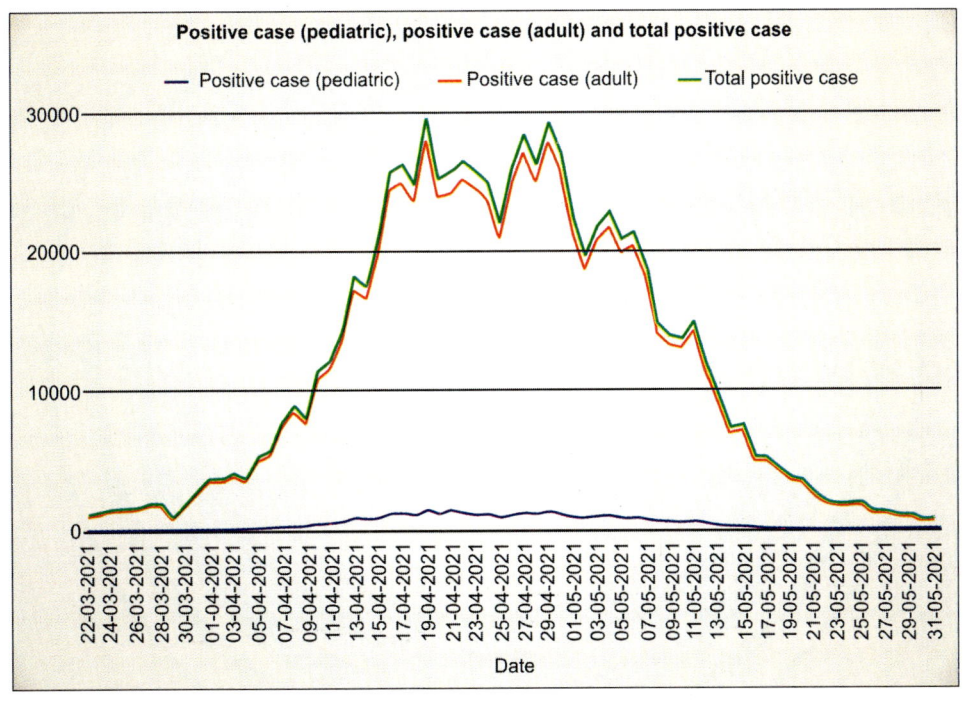

HOSPITALIZATION DATA

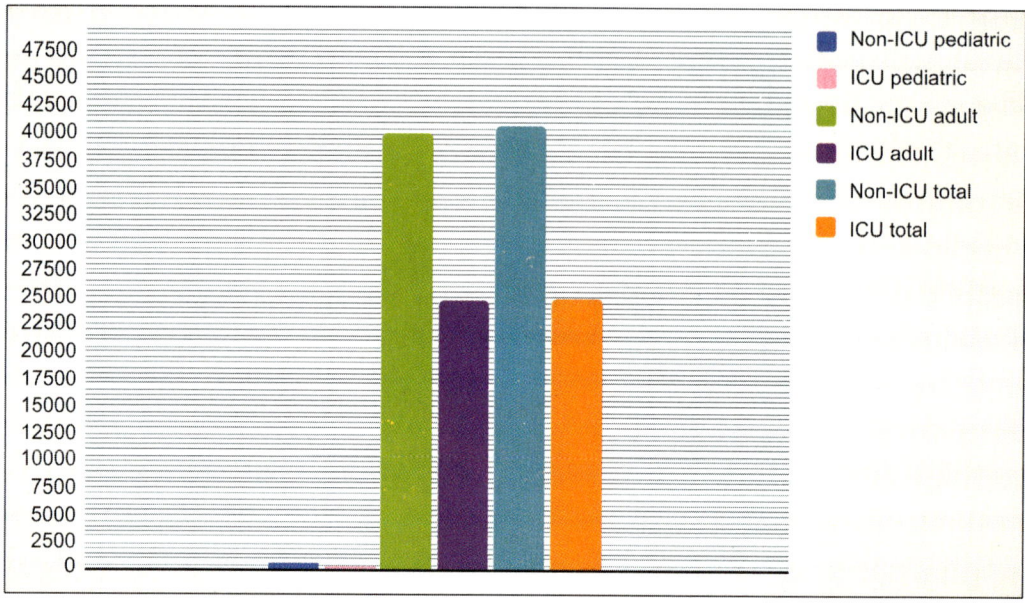

TABLE 13.1: Differences between the first and the second wave of COVID-19 in India		
	First wave	*Second wave*
Causative organism	SARS-Cov-2 virus	Several mutants of SARS-Cov-2 virus
Knowledge about the disease	Less	More
Symptomatology	More related to respiratory system	Newer symptoms like gastrointestinal, etc. adding
Presentation	More severe	Lesser intense
Shortness of breaths	Less cases with breathlessness	More cases with breathlessness
Age profile of the patients	More older population	More younger population
Comorbidities	Patients with comorbidities affected more	Less
Drug availability	Acute shortage and black marketing	Available in the hospitals and pharmacies
Healthcare workers	• Lesser trained people • Fear of acquiring infection • Not vaccinated	• More trained increased • Lesser fear to acquire infections • Mostly vaccinated
Bed capacity	Limited	Enhanced
Ventilator beds	Less than 25000	Increased to more than 50000
Laboratory testing	Only one laboratory in January 2020	More laboratories in private and government center
PPE	Scarcity	Plenty one million PPE produced
Vaccine	Not available	Three approved vaccines available
Treatment affordability	• Increased test price • Increased treatment cost and PPE	• Markedly reduced test price • Reduced treatment cost and PPE

(Contd.)

TABLE 13.1: Differences between the first and the second wave of COVID-19 in India (Contd.)		
	First wave	Second wave
Oxygen requirement to the patient	Less	More
Requirement of mechanical ventilation	Less	More
Disease spread	Slower	Much faster
Plasma therapy	Limited	Much more
Death rate	Higher	Lower
Positivity rate	Lower	Much higher

MUCORMYCOSIS

Mucormycosis, previously called zygomycosis, refers to several different diseases caused by infection with fungi belonging to the order mucorales. Rhizopus species are the most causative organisms of this group. In descending order, the other genera with mucormycosis–causing species include Mucor, Cunninghamella, Apophysomyces, Lichtheimia (formerly Absidia), Saksenaea, Rhizomucor, and other species.

Reasons for increase in mucormycosis in COVID-19 patients:

1. Hyperglycemia due to uncontrolled pre-existing diabetes and high prevalence rates of mucormycosis in India per se.
2. Rampant overuse and irrational use of steroids in management of COVID-19.
3. New onset diabetes due to steroid overuse or severe cases of COVID-19 per se.
4. Prolonged ICU stay and irrational use of broad-spectrum antibiotics.
5. Pre-existing comorbidities, such as hematological malignancies, use of immuno-suppressants, solid organ transplant, etc.
6. Breakthrough infections in patients on voriconazole (anti-fungal drug) prophylaxis.

Signs and Symptoms

1. Facial pain, pain over sinuses, pain in teeth and gums.
2. Paresthesia/decreased sensation over half of face.
3. Blackish discoloration of skin over nasolabial groove/alae nasii.
4. Nasal crusting and nasal discharge which could be blackish or blood tinged.
5. Conjunctival injection or chemosis.
6. Periorbital swelling.
7. Blurring of vision/diplopia.
8. Loosening of teeth/discoloration of palate/gangrenous inferior turbinates.
9. Worsening of respiratory symptoms, hemoptysis, chest pain, alteration of consciousness, headache.

Investigation

i. NCCT PNS (to see bony erosion).
ii. HRCT chest (≥10 nodules, reverse halo sign, CT bronchus sign, etc.) and CT angiography.
iii. MRI brain for better delineation of CNS involvement.

Diagnosis

  i. KOH staining and microscopy, histopathology of debrided tissue and culture.

 ii. MALDI-TOF if available.

iii. Presence of ribbon like aseptate hyphae 5–15 µm that branch at right angles.

Treatment

- One should have a high index of suspicion of invasive fungal infection such as mucormycosis in the presence of predisposing conditions as mentioned above. Timely initiation of treatment reduces mortality. Multidisciplinary team approach is required. Treatment of mucormycosis involves combination of surgical debridement and antifungal therapy.

- Liposomal Amphotericin B in initial dose of 5 mg/kg body weight (10 mg/kg body weight in case of CNS involvement) is the treatment of choice. Each vial contains 50 mg. It should be diluted in 5% or 10% dextrose, it is incompatible with normal saline/ringer lactate. It has to be continued till a favorable response is achieved and disease is stabilized which may take several weeks following which step down to oral Posaconazole (300 mg delayed release tablets twice a day for 1 day followed by 300 mg daily) or Isavuconazole (200 mg 1 tablet 3 times daily for 2 days followed by 200 mg daily) can be done.

- The therapy has to be continued until clinical resolution of signs and symptoms of infection as well as resolution of radiological signs of active disease and elimination of predisposing risk factors, such as hyperglycemia, immunosuppression, etc. it may have to be given for quite long periods of time.

- Conventional Amphotericin B (deoxycholate) in the dose 1–1.5 mg/kg may be used if liposomal form is not available and renal functions and serum electrolytes are within normal limits.

Total number of patients admitted in LNH is: 287.

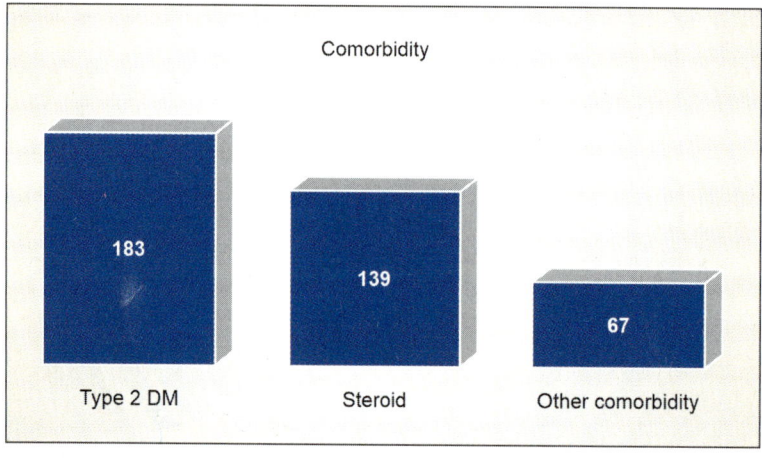

Comorbidity

183 — Type 2 DM

139 — Steroid

67 — Other comorbidity

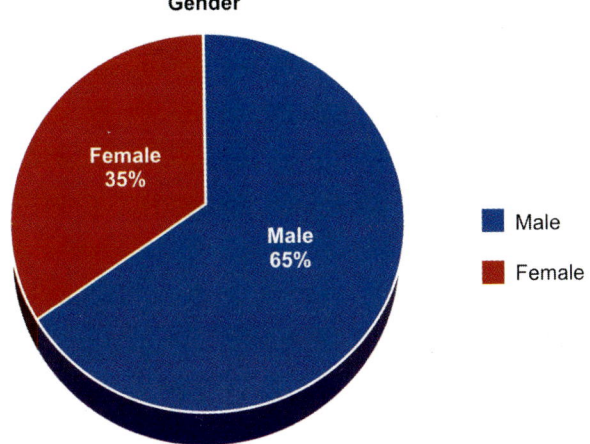

Gender

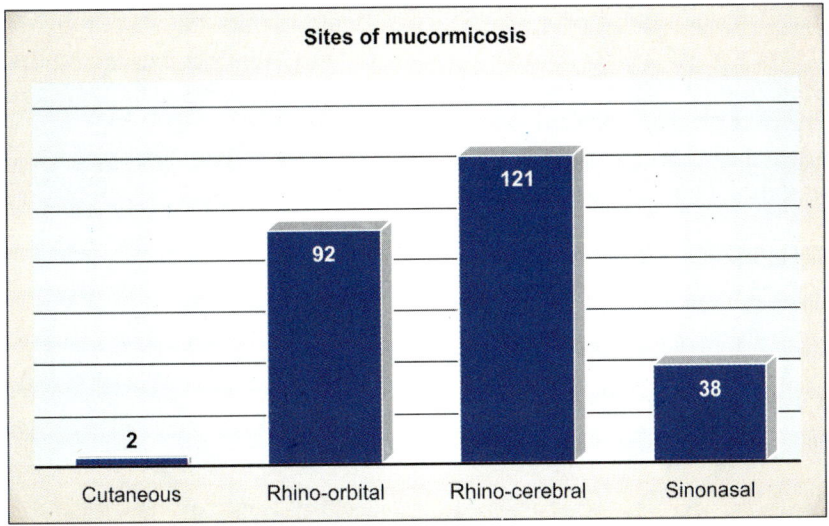

Sites of mucormicosis

Hepatic Manifestation of COVID-19

Suresh Kumar, Harpreet Singh, Rajesh Ruttala

INTRODUCTION

The ongoing pandemic and the research published in the recent year have enhanced the current knowledge about the protean extrapulmonary manifestations of the corona virus.

The presence of ACE 2 receptors in liver cells and biliary tract may be the cause of direct hepatic injury, however it may also be an adverse affects of COVID medications and repurposed drugs commonly being used in COVID.

The pertinent issues of COVID coexistent with hepatic disease and finally vaccination recommendations would be discussed in this chapter.

PATHOGENESIS

SARS-CoV-2 binds to and is internalized into target cells through the angiotensin-converting enzyme 2 (ACE2), which acts as a functional receptor.

ACE2 is present in biliary and liver epithelial cells; therefore, the liver is a potential target for infection (Fig. 14.1).

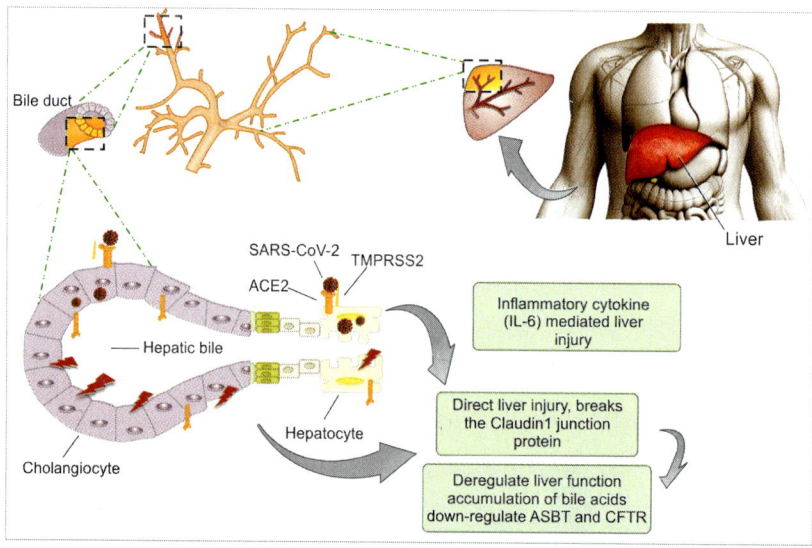

Fig. 14.1: Mechanisms of liver cell and cholangiocyte injury at cellular level

Coronavirus particles have been identified in the cytoplasm of hepatocytes associated with typical histological evidence of viral infection.

MECHANISMS OF HEPATIC INJURY IN COVID-19 (Fig. 14.2)

The elevated liver biochemistries may reflect a direct virus-induced **cytopathic effect** and/or **immune damage** from the provoked inflammatory response and cytokine release syndrome.

The incidence of deranged LFT varies from 14–83% in various series, most common being elevated AST and ALT 1–2 times the upper limit of normal (ULN) and normal to modestly elevated total bilirubin early in the disease process.

Elevations in alkaline phosphatase and gamma glutamyl transferase (GGT) are seen in 6% and 21% of COVID-19 patients, respectively. Liver injury occurs more commonly in severe COVID-19 cases than in mild cases.

Rare cases of severe acute hepatitis and acute liver failure have also been described in patients with COVID-19. Secondary viral infections (HSV) might occur in those treated with corticosteroids and tocilizumab further predisposing to acute liver failure.

In ALF, predictors of peak abnormal liver tests >5 × ULN include age, male gender, body mass index, diabetes mellitus, medications (e.g. lopinavir/ritonavir, hydroxy-chloroquine, remdesivir, tocilizumab), and inflammatory markers (IL-6, ferritin).

Low serum albumin on hospital admission is a marker of COVID-19 severity.

AST is usually higher than ALT and is associated with severe COVID-19 and mortality, which may reflect non-hepatic injury. Baseline liver test abnormalities

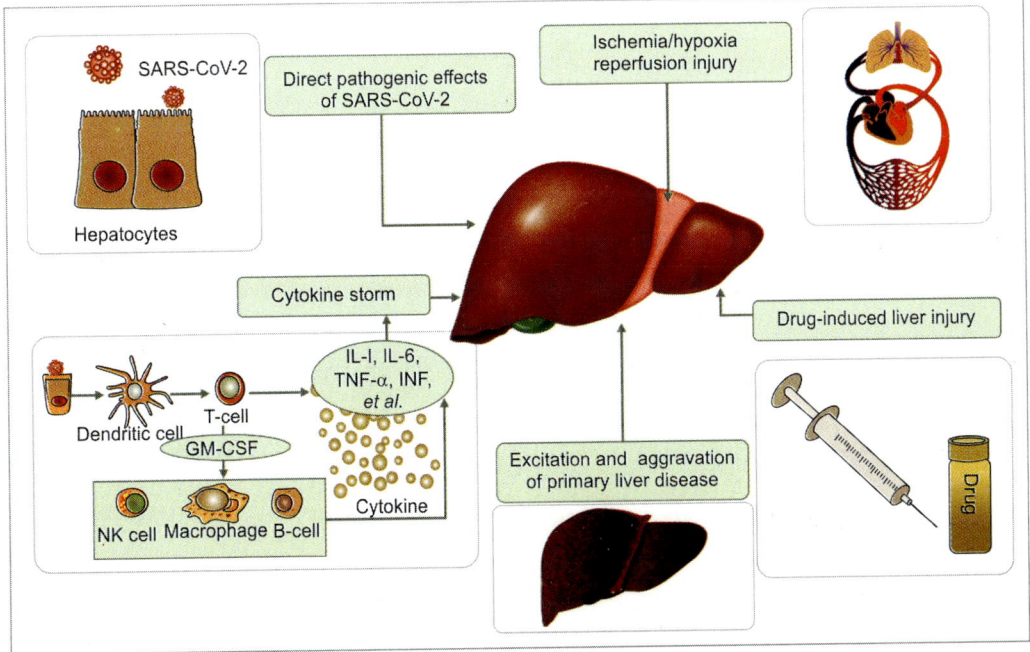

Fig. 14.2: The various mechanisms of hepatic injury in COVID-illustrated

are associated with risk of intensive care unit admission and tend to improve over time.

Alkaline phosphatase peak values are correlated with risk of death and may be predictive of a worse prognosis. Severe liver injury in COVID-19 is uncommon in children; in the rare cases of severe pediatric COVID-19, increases in ALT or AST, when present, are usually mild (<2 × ULN).

Most COVID cases with transient increase in AST and ALT up to 3 times ULN require supportive care and tend to improve over time. In pediatric patients a search for other infective etiology may be required as deranged LFT are uncommon.

Liver histologic assessment from various studies indicate moderate microvesicular steatosis with mild, mixed lobular and portal activity to focal necrosis.

DRUG INDUCED LIVER INJURY (DILI)

Therapeutic agents used to manage symptomatic COVID-19 may be hepatotoxic but rarely require treatment discontinuation. These include remdesivir and tocilizumab.

These drugs might need to be discontinued if AST and ALT rise to 5 × ULN, however due precaution being advised even at levels beyond 3 × ULN, with regular monitoring of LFT and clinical condition.

Overall incidence of DILI is reported around 25%.

Whether SARS-CoV-2 infection exacerbates cholestasis in those with underlying cholestatic liver disease such as primary biliary cholangitis or primary sclerosing cholangitis or with underlying cirrhosis is yet under investigation.

Postmortem studies revealed cholestatic features including bile duct proliferation and canalicular/ductular bile plugs. Secondary sclerosing cholangitis of critically ill patients and cholangiopathy have been reported in some patients with severe COVID-19 and even during recovery.

Differentiating whether increases in liver biochemistries are due to SARS-CoV-2 infection itself; its complications, including myositis (particularly with AST >ALT), cytokine release syndrome, ischemia/hypotension; and/or drug-induced liver injury would be helpful in guiding strategies for patient management individualized to each patient.

HEPATIC VASCULAR EVENTS IN COVID

COVID-19 may predispose patients to thromboembolic disease and anticoagulation may improve outcomes in hospitalized patients.

Acute portal vein thrombosis has been reported in patients with COVID-19; however causality needs to be established. An awareness of the high rate of thrombotic events in COVID-19 is necessary as this could potentially adversely impact the outcomes in those with chronic liver disease.

MORTALITY FROM COVID-19 AND CIRRHOSIS

Mortality in COVID-19 and advanced liver disease higher in more advanced liver disease and strongly associated with hepatic decompensation.

CTP class C conferred a 5 times increased mortality risk as compared to CTP class A patients with COVID.

Acute hepatic decompensation during COVID-19 was strongly associated with subsequent risk of death and almost 21% with acute hepatic decompensation had no respiratory symptoms at presentation. Hepatic decompensation was an independent risk factor for mortality (HR 2.91) in a multicenter, observational US cohort of patients with COVID-19 and cirrhosis.

Alcohol-associated liver disease is a also an independent strong predictor of mortality in COVID-19 and needs to be considered as a significant risk factor at admission.

OUTCOMES IN OTHER HEPATIC DISEASES (HCC, VIRAL HEPATITIS, AIH)

Hepatocellular carcinoma (HCC) is associated with increased all—cause mortality in patients with COVID-19.

Chronic hepatitis B or C (without cirrhosis) have not been associated with mortality from COVID-19.

Interestingly **AIH** (autoimmune hepatitis) patients on immunosuppression did have an increased risk of hospital admission but not ICU admission or risk of death.

The impact of **nonalcoholic fatty liver disease (NAFLD)** on COVID-19 is controversial but metabolic risk factors, such as obesity, diabetes mellitus, and hypertension are associated with COVID-19 severity. NAFLD is associated with progressive COVID-19 and worse outcomes independent of obesity and comorbidities.

The complex decision-making involved in whether or not to proceed with transplantation has been more challenging because of the COVID-19 pandemic. COVID-19 has had a significant impact on the transplant waiting list and transplant center practice patterns.

MANAGEMENT PROTOCOLS SUGGESTED BY AASLD FOR COEXISTENT HEPATIC DISEASES

Treatment for hepatitis B, hepatitis C, AIH, or primary biliary cholangitis (PBC) can be continued if already on treatment.

Viral Hepatitis and AIH

There is no contraindication to initiating treatment of hepatitis B, hepatitis C, AIH, or PBC in patients *without* COVID-19 as clinically warranted. Initiating treatment of hepatitis B in a patient *with* COVID-19 is not contraindicated and should be considered if there is clinical suspicion of a hepatitis B flare or when initiating immunosuppressive therapy **however** initiation of treatment of hepatitis C or PBC in a patient *with* COVID-19 is not routinely warranted and can be deferred until recovered from COVID-19 lowering the overall level of immunosuppression, particularly anti-metabolite dosages (e.g. azathioprine or mycophenolate) based on general principles for managing infections in immunosuppressed patients and to decrease the risk of superinfection is usually beneficial.

A low threshold for considering COVID-19 in patients with new complications for cirrhosis. Acute hepatic decompensation usually warrants testing for SARS-CoV-2.

Usual Drugs Used in COVID

The use of Remdesivir (compensated liver disease) with careful monitoring of LFTs and clinical signs, corticosteroids (dexamethasone doses of 6 mg rather than 8 mg) for those requiring supplemental oxygen and Barcitinab (corticosteroid intolerance) under experimental use, may be followed as per national guidelines. Use of convalescent plasma are unclear as far as outcomes in CLD are concerned.

COVID-19 AND VACCINATION

Vaccination in CLD Patients

The AASLD recommended that patients with CLD who are receiving antiviral therapy for HBV or HCV or medical therapy for primary biliary cholangitis or autoimmune hepatitis should not withhold their medications while receiving the COVID-19 vaccines.

Patients with hepatocellular carcinoma undergoing locoregional or systemic therapy should also be considered for vaccination without interruption of their treatment. However, patients with recent infections or fever should not receive the COVID-19 vaccine until they are medically stable.

mRNA and adenoviral vector COVID-19 vaccines are expected to have a favorable efficacy and safety profile in immunosuppressed patients and may be administered according to their standard dose and schedule. No recommendations for double dosing of these vaccines at present.

Vaccination in Post LT Patients

LT candidates with CLD should receive a COVID-19 vaccine prior to transplantation whenever possible to help ensure an adequate immune response.

CLD patients receiving a COVID-19 vaccine may have local and systemic reactions (fever, myalgias, headache) in the first 48 hours after vaccination. However, respiratory symptoms or systemic symptoms may be indicative of COVID-19 and need further investigations.

The best time to administer the COVID-19 vaccine in liver LT is likely at least 3 months post-LT when immunosuppression is lower and other prophylactic medications are stopped or minimized. However, given the ongoing community spread of SARS-CoV-2, immunization may be initiated as early as 6 weeks post-transplant, especially for the highest-risk individuals with other comorbid factors associated with severe COVID-19.

A reduction in immunosuppression is not recommended in LT recipients solely to elicit an immune response to immunization against SARS-CoV-2 because there is a risk of acute cellular rejection (ACR) with lower immunosuppression.

COVID-19 vaccination may be avoided in LT recipients with active ACR, those being treated for ACR, or those on high daily doses of corticosteroids until the episode is resolved and their baseline immunosuppression reestablished. In patients whose liver tests increase after vaccination and do not immediately return to baseline on repeat testing, a thorough evaluation should follow to exclude ACR or viral infection of the liver.

Given the life saving nature of LT, deceased donor transplantation should not be delayed in a patient who received a COVID-19 vaccine.

If a patient is due for a second dose of an mRNA vaccine in the immediate post-transplant period, this may be delayed 6 weeks to elicit a better immune response.

Potential live liver donors and recipients of live donor livers should be prioritized for COVID-19 vaccination and preferably vaccinated at least two weeks before transplantation when feasible.

However, a lack of COVID-19 vaccination should not delay life saving living donor LT.

Family members and caregivers of LT recipients should be vaccinated against SARS-CoV-2 whenever possible.

BIBLIOGRAPHY

1. AASLD expert panel consensus statement: Vaccines to prevent COVID-19 in patients with liver disease. March 16, 2021.
2. Clinical best practice advice for hepatology and liver transplant providers during COVID-19 pandemic: AASLD expert panel consensus statement. 9 March 2021.
3. Haiyan Wu, et al. Progress in clinical features and pathogenesis of abnormal liver enzymes in Coronavirus disease 2019, Journal of clinical and translational hepatology 2021:9(2),239–46.

Clinical Profile and Management of COVID-19 Infection in Children

Urmila Jhamb, Puneet Kaur Sahi

EPIDEMIOLOGY IN CHILDREN

As per the Indian Union Ministry, till date 8% of the COVID-19 positive cases in India have been children below 17 years of age. In our center (Lok Nayak Hospital, New Delhi), children below 13 years of age comprised 2.6% of the total hospital admissions. Of the admitted children, 20% were treated in PICU/HDU and most of them had comorbidities or coinfections.

CLINICAL FEATURES

Majority of the children who acquire COVID-19 infection are asymptomatic while amongst the symptomatic patients, respiratory and gastrointestinal manifestations make up the commonest reported clinical presentations (Table 15.1). At our hospital, we found that most common symptoms at disease onset were fever, cough, diarrhea, vomiting, irritability and pain abdomen. 11.4% of children developed COVID pneumonia. A small number of cases present as MIS-C (multisystem inflammatory syndrome in children).

TABLE 15.1: Disease severity classification

Clinical severity	Clinical presentation	Clinical parameters
Mild	Symptomatic patients* meeting the case definition for COVID-19	*(Fever, cough, sore throat, fatigue, anorexia, nasal congestion, malaise, headache, diarrhea vomiting, nausea) *without* evidence of viral pneumonia or hypoxia.
Moderate	Pneumonia	Child with clinical signs of pneumonia (cough or difficulty breathing *and* fast breathing *and/or* chest indrawing) *and* no signs of severe pneumonia. Fast breathing (in breaths/min): <2 months: ≥60; 2–11 months: ≥50; 1–5 years: ≥40; 5–10 years: ≥30; 11–18 years: ≥24 While the diagnosis can be made on clinical grounds; chest imaging (radiograph, CT scan, ultrasound) may assist in diagnosis and identify or exclude pulmonary complications.

(Contd.)

TABLE 15.1: Disease severity classification (Contd.)

Clinical severity	Clinical presentation	Clinical parameters
Severe	Severe pneumonia in addition, children with isolated lethargy, seizures, somnolence, diarrhea with severe dehydration are classified in this category	Child with clinical signs of pneumonia *and* at least one of the following: 1. Central cyanosis or SpO_2 <90% 2. Severe respiratory distress (e.g. grunting, very severe chest indrawing) 3. Any of the general danger signs: Inability to breastfeed or drink, lethargy or unconsciousness, or convulsions. Although diagnosis is clinical; chest imaging may provide corroborative evidence and identify or exclude complications.

Critical	Pediatric acute respiratory distress syndrome (PARDS)	PARDS is said to occur in child with *all* of the following:
		1. Acute onset (within 7 days of known clinical insult)
		2. Respiratory failure (not fully explained by cardiac failure or fluid overload) *with*
		3. Chest imaging findings of new infiltrate consistent with acute parenchymal disease *with*
		4. Exclusion of perinatal related lung disease *with*
		5. Oxygenation requirement as **(a)** or **(b)**
		  a. Noninvasive mechanical ventilation:
		    Full face mask bi-level ventilation *or* CPAP ≥5 cm H_2O *with*
		    PaO_2: FiO_2 ratio ≤300 *or* SpO_2: FiO_2 ratio ≤264
		  b. Invasive mechanical ventilation:
		    i. Mild: 4 ≤OI <8 *or* 5 ≤OSI <7.5
		    ii. Moderate: ≤OI <16 *or* 7.5 ≤OSI <12.3
		    iii. Severe: OI ≥16 *or* OSI ≥12.3

	PARDS at risk	PARDS at risk is said to occur in child with *all* of the above points 1 to 4 *with* oxygenation requirement as **(a)** or **(b)** **a. Noninvasive mechanical ventilation** i. Nasal mask CPAP or BiPAP requiring FiO_2 ≤40% to attain SpO_2 of 88–97% ii. Oxygen via mask, nasal cannula or high flow: SpO_2 88–97% with oxygen supplementation at minimal flow Minimal flow <1 year: 2 L/min; 1–5 years: 4 L/min; 5–10 years: 6 L/min; >10 years: 8 L/min **b. Invasive mechanical ventilation:** Oxygen supplementation to maintain SpO_2 ≤88%, but OI <4 *or* OSI <5
	Sepsis	*Suspected or proven infection and ≥2 of 4 age-based systemic inflammatory response syndrome (SIRS) criteria of which one must be **(a)** or **(b)*** a. Abnormal temperature (>38.5°C or <36°C) b. Abnormal white blood cell count for age or >10% bands

(Contd.)

TABLE 15.1: Disease severity classification (Contd.)

Clinical severity	Clinical presentation	Clinical parameters
		c. Tachycardia for age or bradycardia for age if <1 year
		d. Tachypnea for age or need for mechanical ventilation
	Septic shock	Any hypotension (SBP <5th centile or >2 SD below normal forage) corroborating with clinical markers *or* More than two of the following:
		a. Altered mental status
		b. Bradycardia ortachycardia (HR <90 bpm or >160 bpm in infants and heart rate <70 bpmor >150 bpm in children
		c. Prolonged capillary refill (>2 sec) or weak pulse
		d. Mottled or cool peripheries
		e. Reduced urine output

OI (Oxygenation index) = $(FiO_2 \times$ mean airway pressure $\times 100)/PaO_2$.

OSI (Oxygen saturation index) = $(FiO_2 \times$ mean airway pressure $\times 100)/SpO_2$.

MANAGEMENT

Management of Mild Cases

Mild cases need to be isolated to curtail viral transmission either at home, a community facility (COVID care-center) or a health facility (First Referral Units, Community Health Center, sub-district and district hospitals) decided on a case-to-case basis. Prerequisites for home isolation include apt residential conditions for self-isolation and quarantine of family contacts, absence of significant comorbidities and presence of a caregiver with communication link to the hospital.

Persistent high-grade fever beyond 4 days, difficulty in breathing, dip in oxygen saturation <95%, mental confusion, inability to awaken, reduced interaction when awake and inability to drink should prompt urgent referral to a Dedicated COVID Health Center or Hospital.

Mild COVID-19 cases should be given symptomatic treatment with antipyretics, adequate nutrition, and appropriate hydration. Investigations are not required unless there is suspicion for an alternate diagnosis. In children with symptomatic respiratory tract infection, routine use of antibiotics is not recommended except in situations of suspected or confirmed bacterial coinfection. Zinc (0.5–1 mg/kg may be used with maximum of 25–40 mg per day) and vitamin C supplementation (250–500 mg PO OD) may be given for these cases. Available evidence suggests that they reduce inflammatory mediators and enhances microbial killing, although no trials have proven efficacy in COVID-19.

Management of Moderate Cases

Moderate cases should be treated in a Dedicated COVID Health Center or Hospital. All such patients should undergo a detailed clinical history including that of comorbid conditions and for any coexisting infections. Assessment of vital signs, work of breathing and oxygen saturation (SpO_2) is done regularly. Investigations should be done in all cases of moderate to severe/critical COVID-19 as described in Table 15.2.

TABLE 15.2: Investigations in children with moderate to severe COVID-19

Investigation	Rationale	Expected findings
REQUIRED INVESTIGATIONS (should be done)		
Complete blood count (CBC)	Evaluate organ dysfunction	Leucopenia has been reported in 6–26.3% children and lymphopenia in 3.5–40% children
Liver function tests (LFT)	Gauge any complications	Persistent leucopenia, lymphopenia, and thrombocytopenia suggest severe disease
Kidney function test (KFT)	Monitor disease progression	Raised liver transaminases may be seen in one-third children
Chest X-ray (CT thorax is best avoided for diagnostic screening routinely)	Identify COVID-19 pattern and detect other abnormalities	Milder and more focal findings than adults, typically as ground-glass opacities and consolidations with unilateral lower-lobe and peripheral predominance, which regress during recovery time
PREFERRED INVESTIGATIONS (preferably done when available)		
D-dimer Coagulation profile Serum ferritin C reactive protein	To monitor disease severity (including thrombotic risk) and progression To decide anti-coagulation prophylaxis per D-Dimer levels	Raised D-dimer and fibrinogen degradation products (found in 12–17.5% children), ferritin and CRP (found in 13.6% cases) levels are associated with severe disease, cytokine storm and multi-organ dysfunction. Prolongation of aPTT and INR may be seen.
Electrocardiogram (ECG) Echocardiography (ECHO) Cardiac biomarker levels (troponin, CK* and CK MB*)	To rule out cardiac dysfunction in severe COVID-19 cases. To measure corrected QT" (QTc) in patients who start medication that may lead to QT prolongation and arrhythmia like azithromycin	Prolonged PR interval, ST-T segment changes, atrioventricular block, arrhythmia, tachycardia, and low voltage are suggestive of cardiac injury. Raised cardiac enzymes indicate myocarditis or myocardial injury; are associated with severe disease ECHO may identify myocarditis, valvulitis, pericardial effusion, and coronary artery dilatation
DESIRED INVESTIGATIONS (may be done if available)		
LDH levels* Serum IL-6* Serum procalcitonin	Gauge disease severity	Higher IL-6 and LDH levels are shown to correlate with disease severity but not routinely recommended Raised procalcitonin levels may indicate a bacterial coinfection or severe COVID-19 disease while a lower level has a high negative predictive value for a bacterial coinfection

General management should be done as stated above. Additionally, supplemental oxygen therapy may be required for distressed breathing or hypoxia. Empiric antibiotic therapy (in the absence of hypoxia, oral antibiotic like amoxycillin-clavulanic acid/azithromycin; in presence of hypoxia, intravenous ceftriaxone) may be added in under-five children or in case of suspicion of bacterial coinfection. Intravenous fluids should be considered in cases of poor oral acceptance. Corticosteroids may be administered in moderate COVID-19 illness with rapidly progressive disease as detailed below. Close monitoring of patients with moderate COVID-19 is required for signs or symptoms of disease progression.

Management of Severe and Critical Cases

All severe and critical COVID-19 cases should be admitted in a dedicated COVID care hospital.

A detailed history and necessary investigations as described in Table 15.2 are required. Continuous monitoring of vitals, work of breathing and SpO_2 should be done. All patients should be started with intravenous antibiotics (e.g. ceftriaxone) with addition/escalation based on clinical condition or coinfection intravenous fluids should be started and titrated to cardiac status. Corticosteroids should be given for 5–14 days. Anticoagulation and remdesivir may be considered in specific indications as detailed below.

Supplemental oxygen therapy is urgently indicated for any patient with emergency signs (obstructed or absent breathing, severe respiratory distress, central cyanosis, shock, coma or convulsions) or SpO_2 <90%. The most suitable of the following modes of oxygen delivery may be used to provide oxygen to maintain SpO_2 ≤94%:

    I. Conventional oxygen therapy may be given using nasal prongs/cannula, oxygen mask or oxygen hood. Non-rebreathing mask: can provide up to 95% FiO_2 at oxygen flow rate of 10–15 L/min and can be used for short periods only. A triple layer mask may be used to cover the mouth and nose of the patient over the nasal cannula.

    II. HHHFNC/HFNC (heated humidified high flow nasal cannula) may be used in patients who cannot maintain saturation with conventional oxygen therapy. A flow rate of 2L/kg/min can be used up to a maximum of 35 L/min in children and 60 L/min in adults. The FiO_2 can be titrated (21–100%) to the target SpO_2. HFNC has better results than conventional oxygen therapy at the same delivered FiO_2.

    III. Noninvasive ventilation:

        a. *BiPAP (Bilevel Positive Airway Pressure):* It is a form of noninvasive ventilation used in patients with mild acute respiratory distress syndrome without hemodynamic instability, altered mental status or multi-organ failure. However, it has limitations of use in young children as they do not tolerate the oronasal BiPAP mask and become irritable. Only an older and cooperative child can accept BiPAP.

        b. *Bubble CPAP (continuous positive airway pressure):* May be used for newborns and children with severe hypoxemia as an alternative in resource-limited settings.

    IV. Invasive ventilation: Tracheal intubation should be performed when failure of BiPAP occurs or high concentration (FiO_2 >60%) of oxygen is required on HFNC or multiple organ dysfunction occurs. Endotracheal intubation should be performed using airborne precautions. Patients with ARDS, especially young children, may desaturate quickly during intubation.

    Follow rapid sequence intubation with cuffed endotracheal tubes by most experienced person. May use videolaryngoscopy for intubation to maintain safe distance between intubating HCW and patient. Use a plastic sheet to cover the head, neck and chest of patient to minimize contamination. Use disposable ventilator circuits whenever possible. The ARDS protocol for ventilation is used.

Prone ventilation: In resource-limited setting, due to limited availability of HCWs and PPEs, prone ventilation may be difficult to conduct in a child and may unnecessarily increase the risk of infection to the healthcare workers.

ANTIVIRALS, IMMUNOMODULATORS AND OTHER ADJUNCTIVE THERAPIES FOR COVID-19

Steroids are recommended for all patients of severe or critical COVID-19 disease. In moderate COVID-19 disease, steroids should be considered in those with rapid disease progression (progressive deterioration of oxygenation indicators, rapid worsening on imaging and excessive activation of the body's inflammatory response). Dexamethasone 0.15 mg/kg/day (max 6 mg) once a day or methylprednisolone (1–2 mg/kg/day; maximum 80 mg) may be used. Advised duration is 5–14 days based on continuous clinical assessment. These recommendations have been extrapolated from studies conducted mainly in adults.

Anticoagulation: Recommendations for use are moderate to severe COVID with any one of the following:
- D-dimer levels more than 5 times the upper limit of normal.
- One or more non-COVID risk factor for hospital acquired thromboembolism (Central venous catheter, mechanical ventilation, prolonged length of stay, complete immobility, obesity, active malignancy, nephrotic syndrome, cystic fibrosis exacerbation, sickle cell disease, vaso-occlusive crisis, flare of underlying inflammatory disease, congenital or acquired cardiac disease with venous stasis, previous history of VTE, first degree family history of VTE before age 40 years or unprovoked VTE, known thrombophilia, pubertal, postpubertal, or age >12 years, receiving estrogen containing oral contraceptive pill or postsplenectomy for underlying hemoglobinopathy).

Thromboprophylaxis, both mechanical (with sequential compression devices, where feasible) and anticoagulation are recommended. Doses are:

Low molecular weight heparin (enoxaparin): Age < 2 months–1.5 IU/kg/dose SC BD; age >2 months–1 IU/kg/dose SC BD. Unfractionated heparin may be used for children who are clinically unstable or have severe renal impairment as loading dose 75–100 IU/kg intravenous in 10 min followed by initial maintenance dose of 28 IU/kg/hour for age <1 year and 20 IU/kg/hour for 1–18 years (target aPTT between 65–80 seconds). Anticoagulation therapy may be continued till resolution of the hyper-coagulable state or resolution of the clinical risk factors for venous thromboembolism. Thromboprophylaxis is contraindicated in active/major bleeding, need for emergency surgery, platelets <20,000/mm^3, concomitant aspirin administration at doses >5 mg/kg/d and malignant hypertension.

Remdesivir: There are no comparative clinical data evaluating the efficacy or safety of remdesivir for COVID-19 in pediatric patients. Although, initial guidelines contraindicated its use in children <12 years, Emergency Use Authorization (EUA) has been granted for treatment of COVID-19 in hospitalized pediatric patients. In adults, based on available literature, WHO has issued a conditional recommendation against use of remdesivir in COVID-19 while NIH recommends use only in COVID-19 patients with supplemental oxygen requirement where it shortens the time to recovery. It is not routinely recommended in patients on mechanical ventilation as no benefit has been proven at such advanced stage of disease. Few studies in children show promise. The latest guidelines for children recommend use in restricted manner (preferably as part of a clinical trial if available) in moderate to severe COVID-19 with rapidly escalating oxygen need, to be started within 3 days of symptom onset after ruling out contraindications (AST/ALT >5 times upper limit of normal (ULN) and severe renal impairment (eGFR <30 mL/min/m^2 or need for hemodialysis). For children weighing >40 kg, a single loading dose of 200 mg on day 1 followed by once daily dose of 100 mg from day 2 for 5–10 days is used. For children weighing 3.5–40 kg, a single loading dose of 5 mg/kg on day 1 followed by 2.5 mg/kg once daily from day 2 for 5–10 days may be given.

Tocilizumab: Tocilizumab (TCZ), a monoclonal antibody against interleukin-6 (IL-6) receptor has emerged as an alternative treatment for COVID-19 patients with a risk of cytokine storms. While the latest large scale recovery trial suggests benefit of use in hypoxic patients with evidence of systemic inflammation (CRP >75 mg/dl), the proportion of enrolled children is unclear and likely under represented. There are insufficient data to recommend either for or against the use of tocilizumab in hospitalized children. The use of TCZ is suggested only in context of clinical trials in those with moderate/severe disease where oxygen/ventilation requirement is increasing after use of steroids with extensive bilateral lung disease on radioimaging. The dose of TCZ for >30 kg is 8 mg/kg (up to maximum of 800 mg) and <30 kg is 12 mg/kg given as intravenous infusion over 1 hour once, may be repeated if required at 12–24 hours.

Contraindications include use in patients with HIV, those with active infections (uncontrolled systemic bacterial/fungal), tuberculosis, active hepatitis (total bilirubin or AST/ALT raised >5 times ULN), ANC <500–2000/mm^3 and platelet count <50,000–1,00,000/mm^3. Patients should be carefully monitored post Tocilizumab for secondary infections, neutropenia and thrombocytopenia. All patients should obtain a latent tuberculosis (TB) test before TCZ therapy. If the result is positive, TB treatment should be started prior to administration although data from a large number of clinical trials has shown that the risk for latent TB reactivation is very low compared to the benefit of administering TCZ. Safety profile of TCZ in COVID-19 patients is yet to be understood.

Convalescent plasma: Few reports of use of convalescent plasma therapy exist in children with severe COVID-19, leaving uncertainty regarding its safety and efficacy. The latest recovery trial in patients hospitalized with COVID-19, showed that high-titer convalescent plasma did not improve survival or other prespecified clinical outcomes.

Other Agents for COVID-19

There is no role of azithromycin, hydroxychloroquine, choloroquine, favipiravir, lopinavir/ritonavir, umifenovir in children with COVID-19. There is insufficient evidence for or against use of ivermectin in children with COVID except in context of clinical trials. Multiple potential treatments are under evaluation including interferon-beta, anti-IL-6 receptor monoclonal antibodies (sarilumab), anti-IL-6 monoclonal antibody (siltuximab), Bruton's tyrosine kinase inhibitors, acalabrutinib, ibrutinib, zanubrutinib) and Janus kinase inhibitors (baricitinib, ruxolitinib, tofacitinib). However, there is insufficient data for recommending use of any of these agents in children except in the context of a clinical trial.

MULTISYSTEM INFLAMMATORY SYNDROME IN CHILDREN (MIS-C)

WHO Criteria for Diagnosis of MIS-C

Children and adolescents 0–19 years of age with fever $\geq$3 days.
AND two of following:
1. Rash or bilateral non-purulent conjunctivitis or mucocutaneous inflammation signs (oral, hands or feet).
2. Hypotension or shock.
3. Features of myocardial dysfunction, pericarditis, valvulitis, or coronary abnormalities (including ECG, ECHO findings or elevated troponin/NT-pro BNP).
4. Evidence of coagulopathy (by PT, PTT, elevated d-dimers).
5. Acute gastrointestinal problems (diarrhea, vomiting, or abdominal pain).
AND
Elevated markers of inflammation such as ESR, C-reactive protein, or procalcitonin.
AND
No other obvious microbial cause of inflammation, including bacterial sepsis, staphylococcal or streptococcal shock syndromes.
AND
Evidence of COVID-19 (RT-PCR, antigen test or serology positive), or likely contact with patients with COVID-19.

Investigations

A tiered diagnostic approach (Tier 1 followed by 2) is recommended in patients *without life-threatening manifestations* which includes performing an initial screening evaluation (Tier 1), and proceeding to a complete diagnostic work-up (Tier 2) only in patients with laboratory results from the Tier 1 screening that are concerning (i.e. elevated ESR >40 mm/hr. and/or CRP >5 mg/dl and at least 1 other suggestive laboratory feature: lymphopenia (ALC <1000/mm,^{3} neutrophilia, thrombocytopenia, hyponatremia, or hypoalbuminemia) and after ruling out possible coinfections/alternate diagnosis. However, in sick children, both Tier 1 and 2 investigations as well as investigation to rule out coinfections go hand-in-hand.

Tier 1 investigations: CBC, KFT, LFT, SE, blood glucose, blood gas, ESR, CRP and testing for SAR-CoV-2 by RT-PCR or serology*

Tier 2 investigations: Coagulation profile (PT, aPTT, D-dimer, fibrinogen), inflammatory markers (ferritin, LDH, procalcitonin, triglycerides, IL-6) cardiac markers (electrocardiogram, ECHO, BNP, troponin T).

---

*Diagnosis of MISC essentially requires ruling out any possible coinfection or alternate cause of symptoms. Therefore, it is recommended to specifically work-up for tropical infections like dengue, malaria, enteric fever, leptospira and scrub typhus and shock syndromes like (streptococcal and staphyloccal toxic shock syndromes) along with Tier 1 investigations.

Treatment

Hospitalized children of MISC with life-threatening manifestations (shock, coronary dilation, MODS):

a. Admit in PICU, start intravenous fluids, give respiratory and inotropic support as indicated and monitor continuously.

b. Immunomodulatory therapy
  i. Administer intravenous immunoglobulin (IVIG) (total dose 2 gm/kg; maximum 100 gm) over 1–2 days).
  ii. Add low dose glucocorticoids. Start with intravenous methylprednisolone—1–2 mg/kg/day once a day for 3–5 days, then shift to oral methylprednisolone or equivalent dose of dexamethasone. These are to be tapered and stopped over 3–4 weeks with 25% reduction per week with serial laboratory and cardiac assessment.
  iii. If unresponsive to above (persistent fevers and/or significant end-organ involvement despite initial immunomodulatory treatment), consider high dose steroids (intravenous methylprednisolone 10–30 mg/kg/day for 3–5 days) and/or second dose of IVIG. ACR guidelines recommends high dose steroids over IVIG due to higher risk of complications with the latter in these patients.
  iv. If still unresponsive to above, may consider high dose Anakinra; 2–10 mg/kg/dose (max 100 mg/dose) SC/IV q6–12h or infliximab (>6 years old) 5 mg/kg IV.

c. Anti-coaguulation and antiplatelet therapy
  i. Aspirin (3–5 mg/kg/day up to 81 mg once daily) is recommended in all MIS-C patients without active bleeding or significant bleeding risk. It should be continued until normalization of platelet count and confirmed normal coronary arteries at ≥4 weeks after diagnosis.
  ii. Anticoagulation with enoxaparin (factor Xa level 0.5–1.0) or warfarin in MIS-C patients with a coronary artery z-score greater than 10.0 or LVEF <35% is advised.

d. Start on initial broad-spectrum antibiotics considering symptom overlap with severe bacterial infection.

In children of MISC without life-threatening manifestations: Investigations to rule out other possible etiologies should be done before initiating immunomodulatory therapy (ACR). IVIG should be administered as described above. Glucocorticoids may also be added to IVIG as first-line therapy in patients who have not yet developed shock or severe end-organ involvement but present with concerning features such as ill appearance, highly elevated BNP, or unexplained tachycardia.

All children with MIS-C require ongoing clinical monitoring while laboratory investigations may be repeated every 24–48 hourly as guided by the clinical condition. For children with cardiac involvement, repeat ECG 48 hourly and ECHO at 7–14 days and between 4 to 6 weeks (and after 1 year, if initial ECHO was abnormal).

In our experience, working in one of the largest tertiary care COVID hospitals of Delhi, with nearly 450 pediatric COVID admissions till date, MIS-C was diagnosed in an exceedingly small number of patients.

MANAGEMENT OF NEONATES BORN TO COVID-19 POSITIVE MOTHERS

Standard neonatal resuscitation measures should be followed with positive pressure ventilation delivered by self-inflating bag and mask rather than a T piece resuscitator, if needed. If the baby requires intensive care, a single patient room with negative pressure is preferred. The baby should be tested at 24 hours of life. Neonates with COVID-19 are mostly asymptomatic, a small proportion present with *nonspecific* signs, symptoms and laboratory and radiological findings. Asymptomatic positive babies should be re-tested on day 5 and discharged if negative. If positive on day 5, lack of any symptoms till day 10 qualifies for discharge.

The mother-baby dyad should not be separated unless mother is critically sick. It is critical that breastfeeding should be encouraged within 1 hour of birth with the mother wearing a mask and following meticulous hand hygiene as benefits of breastfeeding far outweigh the risks of transmission. Rooming-in, and kangaroo mother care should go on as usual. If the mother is unable to room-in due to sickness, her baby may be fed using expressed milk. The baby should be vaccinated prior to discharge from the hospital. All these recommendations are applicable to preterm as well as low birth weight babies.

DISCHARGE CRITERIA AND FOLLOW-UP

The patient with mild to moderate disease can be discharged after 10 days of symptom onset and no fever or oxygen requirement for 3 consecutive days and complete resolution of symptoms prior to discharge. There will be no need for RT-PCR testing before discharge. Patient should home quarantine for another 7 days post discharge. For those with severe disease and immunocompromised states (like cancer transplant recipients and HIV) should not only have complete resolution of symptoms but also a documented negative RT-PCR test report prior to discharge.

BIBLIOGRAPHY

1. Agarwal A, Basmaji J, Muttalib F, et al. High-flow nasal cannula for acute hypoxemic respiratory failure in patients with COVID-19: systematic reviews of effectiveness and its risks of aerosolization, dispersion, and infection transmission. Les canules nasales à haut débit pour le traitement de l'insuffisance respiratoire hypoxémique aiguë chez les patients atteints de la COVID-19: comptes rendus systématiques de l'efficacité et des risques d'aérosolisation, de dispersion et de transmission de l'infection. *Can J Anaesth.* 2020;67(9):1217–48.
2. Chiotos K, Hayes M, Kimberlin DW, et al. Multicenter Interim Guidance on Use of Antivirals for Children With Coronavirus Disease 2019/Severe Acute Respiratory Syndrome Coronavirus 2. *J Pediatric Infect Dis Soc.* 2021;10(1):34–48. doi:10.1093/jpids/piaa115
3. Clinical management of COVID-19. Interim guidance. WHO. Published 27 May 2020. Available at: https://www.who.int/publications/i/item/clinical-management-of-covid-19. Last accessed on 18 Sept, 2020.
4. Coronavirus in India: 54 pc COVID-19 cases in age group 18-44 years, 51 pc deaths among those aged 60 years and above. Published Sep 02, 2020. Available at:https:/www.financialexpress.com/lifestyle/health/coronavirus-in-india-54-pc-covid-19-cases-in-age-group-18-44-years-51-pc-deaths-among-those-aged-60-years-and-above/2072525/. Last accessed 18 Sept 2020.
5. Dong Y, Mo X, Hu Y, et al. Epidemiology of COVID-19 Among Children in China. *Pediatrics.* 2020;145(6):e20200702.
6. Goldenberg NA, Sochet A, Albisetti M, et al. Consensus-based clinical recommendations and research priorities for anticoagulant thromboprophylaxis in children hospitalized for COVID-19-related illness. J Thromb Haemost. 2020;18:3099–105.
7. Goldman DL, Aldrich ML, Hagmann SHF, et al. Compassionate Use of Remdesivir in Children With Severe COVID-19. *Pediatrics.* 2021;147(5):e2020047803.doi:10.1542/peds.2020–047803

8. Henderson LA, Canna SW, Friedman KG, et al. American College of Rheumatology Clinical Guidance for Multisystem Inflammatory Syndrome in Children Associated With SARS-CoV-2 and Hyperinflammation in Pediatric COVID-19: Version 2. *Arthritis Rheumatol.* 2021;73(4):e13-e29. doi:10.1002/art.41616)

9. IAP (Indian academy of pediatrics) advanced life support course provider manual 2015 (page 160–1).

10. IAP COVID-19 management guidelines April 2021. Avaialable from: https://iapindia.org/pdf/yOQBzDmtbU4R05M_IAP%20Covid%2019%20managementGuidelines%20for%20Pediatrician%20V1.1%20Apr%2027_2021%20(2).pdf. Published April 2021. Last accessed 01 June, 2021.

11. Ministry of Health and Family Welfare Government of India Protocol for Management of COVID-19 in the Paediatric Age Group. Available from: https://www.mohfw.gov.in/pdf/Protocol for Management of COVID-19 in the Paediatric Age Group.pdfPublished 20 april 2021. Last accessed 01 June 2021.

12. NIH COVID-19 Treatment Guidelines. Special considerations in children. Available from: https://www.covid19treatmentguidelines.nih.gov/special-populations/children/. Last updated 21 april 2021. Last accessed 01 June 2021.

13. Pediatric Acute Lung Injury Consensus Conference Group. Pediatric acute respiratory distress syndrome: consensus recommendations from the Pediatric Acute Lung Injury Consensus Conference. Pediatr Crit Care Med 2015;16:428–39.

14. Recovery Collaborative Group, Horby P, Lim WS, et al. Dexamethasone in Hospitalized Patients with COVID-19—Preliminary Report [published online ahead of print, 2020 Jul 17]. N Engl J Med. 2020;NEJMoa2021436.

15. Recovery Collaborative Group. Convalescent plasma in patients admitted to hospital with COVID-19 (recovery): a randomised controlled, open-label, platform trial [published online ahead of print, 2021 May 14]. *Lancet.* 2021;S0140-6736(21)00897-7. doi:10.1016/S0140-6736(21)00897-7).

16. Recovery Collaborative Group. Tocilizumab in patients admitted to hospital with COVID-19 (recovery): a randomised, controlled, open-label, platform trial. *Lancet.* 2021;397(10285):1637–45. doi:10.1016/S0140-6736(21)00676-0

17. Revised Discharge Policy for COVID-19. Government of India. Ministry of health and family welfare. Published on 8 May, 2020. Available at: https://www.mohfw.gov.in/pdf/ReviseddischargePolicyforCOVID19.pdf. Last accessed 18 Sept, 2020.

18. Revised guidelines for Home Isolation of very mild/pre-symptomatic/asymptomatic COVID-19 cases. Government of India Ministry of Health and Family Welfare. Published July 2, 2020. Available at: https://www.mohfw.gov.in/pdf/RevisedHomeIsolationGuidelines.pdf. Last accessed on 18 Sep, 2020.

19. Sahi PK, Jhamb U, Dabas A. Pediatric Coronavirus Disease 2019: Clinical Features and Management. *Indian Pediatr.* 2021;58(5):453–60. doi:10.1007/s13312-021-2216-4

20. Sundaram M, Ravikumar N, Bansal A, et al. Novel Coronavirus 2019 (2019-nCoV) Infection: Part II–Respiratory Support in the Pediatric Intensive Care Unit in Resource-limited Settings. *Indian Pediatr.* 2020;57(4):335–42.

21. Updated Clinical Management Protocol for COVID-19. Ministry of health and family welfare. Government of India. Published July 3, 2020. Available at: https://www.mohfw.gov.in/pdf/Updated Clinical Management Protocol for COVID 19 dated 03072020.pdf. Last accessed August 3, 2020.

22. World Health Organisation. Therapeutics and COVID-19: living guideline. Available from https://www.who.int/publications/i/item/WHO-2019-nCoV therapeutics-2021.1. Published on 31 March 2021. Last accessed 01 June 2021.

23. Zaffanello M, Piacentini G, Nosetti L, Franchini M. The use of convalescent plasma for pediatric patients with SARS-CoV-2: A systematic literature review. *Transfus Apher Sci.* 2021;60(2):103043. doi:10.1016/j.transci.2020.103043.

COVID-19 and Cardiovascular Manifestations: Indian Perspectives

Bhushan Shah, Mohit D Gupta, Shekhar Kunal, Girish MP

INTRODUCTION

Coronavirus disease 2019 (COVID-19), caused by a severe acute respiratory syndrome coronavirus 2 (SARS-CoV-2), was first documented in Wuhan, China in December 2019. Within a span of three months owing to its rapid spread, WHO declared COVID-19 as a global pandemic. This rapid spread is largely due to its high infectivity, prolonged asymptomatic phase and uninterrupted global travel. India is currently witnessing a severe second wave of the pandemic with a huge disease burden with 27,729,247 confirmed cases of COVID-19 and accounting for 322,512 deaths. COVID-19 infection has a multisystem involvement with respiratory and cardiovascular (CV) system being predominantly affected in most of the patients. A majority of CV complications occur within the first or second week of presentation. The spectrum of CV involvement in acute COVID-19 infection includes acute cardiac injury, myocarditis, acute coronary syndrome (ACS), cardiac arrhythmias, heart failure, cardiogenic shock and venous thromboembolism (VTE). CV manifestations are also known to occur post resolution of acute COVID-19 illness and is termed "post COVID-19 syndrome".

EPIDEMIOLOGY

SARS-CoV-2, a member of the Coronaviridae family is an enveloped virus with non-segmented, single stranded, positive-sense RNA genome. It is believed that SARS-CoV-2 has originated from bats to an intermediate host and finally to humans. This novel coronavirus infection is marked by a rapid person to person spread with median incubation period of about 5 days. SARS-CoV-2 infection is caused by binding of the viral surface spike protein to the human angiotensin-converting enzyme 2 (ACE2) receptor following activation of the spike protein by transmembrane protease serine 2 (TMPRSS2). ACE2 receptor are predominantly expressed on type II pneumocytes in the lungs, heart, intestine, kidneys and blood vessels. Following binding to the receptors, SARS-CoV-2 enters the cells via receptor-mediated endocytosis, followed by synthesis of viral proteins and genetic material, and subsequent release of mature virions by exocytosis. However, most of the pathogenic effects of COVID-19 occurs as a result of the heightened inflammatory response following SARS-CoV-2 infection. Multisystem involvement in COVID-19 is mediated by multiple inflammatory cytokines leading to a cytokine storm and end organ damage. The viral RNA serves as the major pathogenic molecule recognized by the cells of the innate immune response thereby activating multiple inflammatory cells. This results in production of IFN-α/β and other pro-inflammatory molecules such as IL-1, IL-2, IL-4, IL-6, IL- 10, IL-12, GCSF, IFN-γ and TNF-α. This massive production of cytokines leads to increased vascular permeability, alveolar epithelial damage, ARDS and multisystem involvement.

CARDIOVASCULAR COMORBIDITIES AND OUTCOME IN COVID-19

Cardiovascular risk factors and cardiovascular diseases (CVD) are common comorbidity in patients with COVID-19. These patients are more vulnerable to severe COVID-19 infection as well as its sequelae with worse clinical outcomes. In a large study from China studying clinical characteristics of 1,099 patients with COVID-19 reported that 24% had CV comorbidity, with HTN in 15%, DM in 7.4%, and coronary heart disease in 2.4%. Similarly a meta-analysis involving eight studies from china including 46,248 COVID-19 patients showed the most prevalent comorbidities was hypertension (HTN) (17 ± 7%, 95% CI 14–22%) and diabetes mellitus (DM) (8 ± 6%, 95% CI 6–11%), followed by CVDs (5 ± 4%, 95% CI 4–7%). The odds of hypertension (OR: 2.36, 95% CI: 1.46–3.83) and CVDs (OR: 3.42, 95% CI: 1.88–6.22) were higher in severe patients as compared to non-severe group. In one of the largest series of 44,762 confirmed COVID-19 patients, comorbidities such as HTN was reported in 12.8%, DM in 5.3% and CVDs in 4.2% subjects. The case fatality rate (CFR) were higher among patients with comorbidities such as CVD (10.5%), diabetes (7.3%) and hypertension (6%) as compared to overall case-fatality rate of 2.3%. Potential explanations for susceptibility and increasing severity of COVID-19 infection in patients with pre-existing CVDs include CVD being more prevalent in those with advancing age with a functionally dysregulated immune system and higher expression of ACE2. Thus, prevalent CVD may be a marker of accelerated immunologic aging/dysregulation and relates indirectly to COVID-19 outcome.

CARDIOVASCULAR SPECTRUM OF COVID-19 (Fig. 16.1)

Acute Myocardial Injury

Acute myocardial injury is defined as "elevation of high-sensitivity cardiac troponin (hs-cTn) above the 99th percentile of its upper limit of normal or evidence of new electrocardiographic (ECG) or echocardiographic abnormalities". One of the earliest evidence of acute myocardial injury in COVID-19 came from a series of 138 COVID-19 hospitalized patients from Wuhan China wherein it was reported in 7.2% (10/138) of patients. In the same series, among the critically ill patients, acute cardiac injury was documented in 22% suggesting a more severe illness. Data from India is restricted to a small retrospective study wherein 25.9% (28/108) patients had acute cardiac injury, especially those with cardiovascular comorbidities, such as hypertension, coronary artery disease and diabetes. A large meta-analysis of 1,527 COVID-19 patients revealed that 8% of them had acute myocardial injury with the risk of myocardial injury being 13-fold higher in patients with severe illness. The etiology of COVID-19 induced acute myocardial injury is often thought to be varied with plaque rupture, thrombosis (type I MI) or supply-demand mismatch (type II MI), disseminated intravascular coagulation (DIC), and non-ischemic injury such as myocarditis, stress-induced cardiomyopathy,

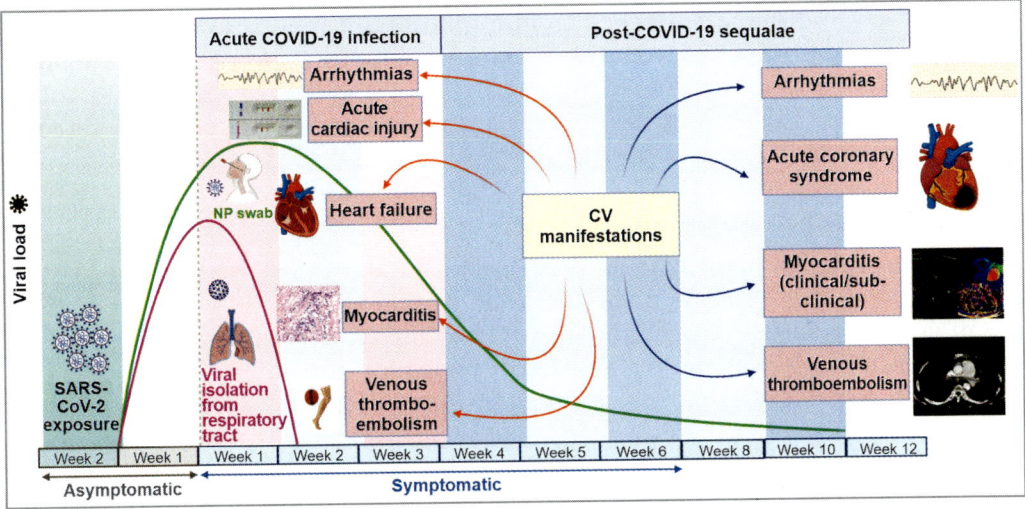

Fig. 16.1: Central illustration: Spectrum of cardiovascular manifestation in COVID-19

cytokine release syndrome, acute pulmonary embolism being the plausible hypotheses. Each of this results from either direct or indirect effect of severe viral infection. Evidence from studies on COVID-19 infected patients indicates two different pattern of acute myocardial injury. The first pattern reflects a delayed occurrence often noted during 2nd or 3rd week of illness and is often related to cytokine storm, severe hypoxemia due to respiratory failure rather than isolated direct myocardial injury. In contrast, another pattern of acute cardiac injury presents acutely with predominant cardiac symptoms suggesting viral myocarditis (direct injury) or stress cardiomyopathy. There is a need to differentiate between these two patterns as the latter responds dramatically to intravenous immunoglobulin and steroids.

Myocarditis

Myocarditis can be an initial presentation of COVID-19 which may be either focal or global myocardial inflammation. Its exact pathogenesis is still unclear. There is a paucity of literature on the incidence of COVID-19 induced myocarditis. In a retrospective multicenter study from China, among the 68 deaths of patients with laboratory-confirmed COVID-19 infection, 7% were attributed to myocarditis with circulatory failure and in 33% of cases myocarditis played a contributing role in patient's death. Two case reports of fulminant myocarditis in a COVID-19 patient with no underlying cardiovascular disease were reported from China with both of them improving with antiviral therapy, intravenous corticosteroids, immunoglobulins, ionotropic support and extracorporeal membrane oxygenation (ECMO). Most of the diagnosis of myocarditis in COVID-19 are based on clinical, ECG findings, elevated cardiac enzymes supported by echocardiographic/cardiac magnetic resonance (CMR) imaging evidence and normal coronaries on angiogram. In a CMR based study from Germany involving 100 COVID-19 recovered middle aged adults, a high prevalence of myocarditis (60%) was reported. This was independent of the pre-existing conditions, severity, overall course of the acute illness and time from the original diagnosis. In another CMR based study among 145 competitive student athletes who had recovered from mild to moderate COVID-19 illness without requiring hospitalization, a low prevalence of myocarditis 1.4% (2/145) was reported. Such variations have led to a lack of understanding about the true incidence of myocarditis in COVID-19. Since endomyocardial biopsy was not carried out in most of these patients, our understanding of the disease process is limited.

Acute Coronary Syndrome (ACS)

COVID-19 infection in patients with significant CV risk factors, or established CVD, have led to likely rise in incidence of ACS in the setting of SARS-CoV-2 infection. The true prevalence is often underreported owing to limited testing and availability of cardiac catheterization laboratory. This led to a significant challenge in managing CV emergencies with COVID-19. It is essential to differentiate ACS from its mimics in order to provide adequate treatment and avoid risks. In a study analyzing the impact of COVID-19 on STEMI care, there was a significant increase in time components such as symptom onset to first medical contact (FMC), door to device and catheterization laboratory arrival to device time. The most plausible explanation for this delay was that patients were hesitant to visit a hospital during the pandemic leading to a pre-hospital delay or seeking no care at all. This critical time delay in the hospital was also attributed to detailed evaluation in the emergency department prior to shifting to catheterization laboratories, infection control measures including patient preparation and time consumed in wearing personal protective gears. In a study from India during COVID 19 pandemic, there was 43% decline in the AMI admissions with most of them having delayed presentation as evident by the prolongation of symptom to door time. This delayed presentation was probably responsible for the low LV ejection fraction (LVEF) noted in these patients on admission. They also noted a subsequent increase in duration of hospital stay and cardiac medications on discharge attributed to lower LVEF. In order to slowdown the COVID-19 pandemic, lockdown was enforced globally as well as in India which led to unintentional change in acute cardiovascular care. Currently, a multicentric CSI-AMI study from India evaluating AMI admissions patterns as well as rates of thrombolysis/primary percutaneous intervention, changes in the major complications and mortality rates of AMI is underway which will guide formation of future guidelines to improve acute cardiovascular care in India. Chinese, American and European CV associations have published position statements and recommendations for optimal management of patients with ACS during COVID-19 pandemic with marked differences as highlighted in Tables 16.1 and 16.2.

Heart Failure (HF) and Cardiogenic Shock

New or existing HF in the setting of COVID-19 can complicate presentation, management, and prognosis of COVID-19 patients. In an initial study from Wuhan, China, HF was reported in 4.1% (17/416) of the COVID-19 population. In contrast to this, another study from China, reported HF in 44/191 (23%) patients with a significant proportion of non-survivors having HF (52% *vs* 21%; p <0.001). It remains unclear whether the HF is possibly due to exacerbation of pre-existing left ventricular dysfunction or new onset cardiomyopathy (either due to myocarditis or stress cardiomyopathy). The etiology of COVID-19 induced HF is multifactorial. The proposed hypothesis includes (a) virus-induced infiltration of inflammatory cells

TABLE 16.1: STEMI recommendations: Fibrinolysis versus PCI

Peking Union Medical College Hospital (China) recommendation

1. STEMI patients with suspected or confirmed COVID-19 infection presenting within 12 hours of symptoms onset should undergo strict isolation followed by thrombolysis if no contraindication exists.
2. Based on SARS-CoV-2 testing result status after thrombolysis patient may be transferred to a designated infectious medical institution or cardiac care unit.
3. STEMI patients presenting out of window period with ongoing symptoms, hemodynamic instability, arrhythmias or contraindication for thrombolysis or failed thrombolysis, should undergo risk versus benefit evaluation followed by catheterization with proper personal protective equipment (PPE).

ACC/SCAI joint statement

1. STEMI patient with confirmed COVID-19 infection, balance between healthcare workers (HCWs) exposure and patient benefit will need to be weighed carefully.
2. Fibrinolysis can be considered for a relatively stable STEMI patient with active COVID-19 infection.
3. STEMI patient with active COVID-19 infection in whom primary percutaneous coronary intervention (PCI) is considered then it should be done wearing proper PPE.

European association of percutaneous cardiovascular interventions (EAPCI) position statement

1. Invasive coronary angiography for COVID-19-positive patients with elevation in hs-cTn should be restricted to those with type 1 MI.
2. Timely reperfusion of STEMI patients should not be compromised during COVID 19 pandemic. Reperfusion strategy as per current guidelines should be preferred in patients with onset of symptoms of ischemia <12 hours duration and persistent ST-segment elevation in at least two contiguous ECG leads.
3. In the absence of rapid SARS-CoV-2 testing, all STEMI patients should be considered as COVID-19 positive and managed accordingly to ensure safety of healthcare workers (HCWs).
4. All STEMI patients should undergo SARS-CoV-2 testing as soon as possible following first medical contact (FMC) irrespective of reperfusion strategy, at the latest upon admission to the ICU post primary PCI. Until the test result are available, all precautionary measures to avoid potential infection of other patients and HCWs should be implemented.
5. The maximum delay from STEMI diagnosis to reperfusion therapy should not exceed 120 minutes.
6. Primary PCI should be the first line therapy of reperfusion if feasible within 120 minutes time frame. It should only be performed in facilities approved for the treatment of COVID-19 patients so that safety of HCWs and other patients can be assured.
7. Fibrinolysis if not contraindicated should be first line of therapy. If the target time of 120 minutes cannot be met. Fibrinolysis should only be undertaken if type 1 MI is highly likely.
8. Complete revascularization should be done during the same hospitalization if indicated and appropriate in order to avoid staged procedures which would need readmissions and re-exposure during the ongoing crisis.
9. Evaluation of left ventricular (LV) function in patients undergoing invasive revascularization should be done with LV angiography.

TABLE 16.2: NSTEACS recommendation: Invasive versus conservative

Peking Union Medical College Hospital (China) recommendations

1. Low/intermediate risk NSTEMI and hemodynamically stable to undergo medical therapy PCI post COVID-19 treatment.
2. Very high and high-risk NSTEMI patients, risk versus benefit assessment to be done followed by PCI with strict isolation.

ACC/SCAI joint statement

1. NSTEMI with suspected COVID-19 infection timing should allow for SARS-CoV-2 testing prior to cardiac catheterization for a more informed decision regarding infection control.
2. Rapid discharge of patients following revascularization for maximizing bed availability and reducing patient exposure within the hospital. Follow-up through teleconsultation should be done in most cases.
3. Low/intermediate risk NSTEMI patients with known COVID-19 conservative therapy may be sufficient.
4. Unstable patients with NSTEMI may be considered for PCI after adequate PPE measures.

EAPCI position statement

1. Management of patients with non-ST-segment elevation ACS (NSTE-ACS) should be guided by risk stratification.
2. All NSTE-ACS patients should undergo SARS-CoV-2 testing as early as possible following FMC, irrespective of treatment strategy.
3. Risk stratification should be based on the criteria published by ESC guidelines on NSTE-ACS. It is slightly modified in view of infection control. GRACE scoring is excluded. Patients should be categorized into four risk groups, i.e. very high-risk, high-risk, intermediate risk, and low-risk and managed accordingly.
4. Very high-risk NSTE-ACS patients should be managed similar to STEMI.
5. High-risk NSTE-ACS patients should receive medical therapy for stabilization and prompt SARS-CoV-2 testing is recommended, while an early (<24 hours) invasive strategy is planned. The time of the invasive strategy may be prolonged (>24 hours) according to the availability of test results.
6. Intermediate risk NSTEACS patients should receive medical therapy for stabilization and prompt SARS-CoV-2 testing is recommended. Patients should be carefully evaluated for alternative diagnosis which mimics as ACS. If an alternative diagnosis is considered a noninvasive testing with CCTA should be favored. At this times of high demand on the infrastructure and reduced availability of catheterization labs and/or operators, noninvasive conservative management with early discharge from the hospital and planned clinical follow-up should be considered.
7. Low-risk NSTEACS patients should receive conservative strategy based on noninvasive testing. CCTA protocol should be added to CT thorax scan performed in COVID 19 patients.

impairing the myocardial function, (b) pro-inflammatory state/cytokine storm leading to necrosis and death of the myocardium predisposing to stress cardiomyopathy and cytokine-related myocardial dysfunction, (c) endothelial injury coupled with micro-thrombosis leading to endocardial damage, (d) ARDS and respiratory failure culminating in heart failure due to severe hypoxia by causing imbalance between supply of oxygen and the higher demand of the myocardium. Right heart failure and associated pulmonary hypertension occurs in patients with severe parenchymal lung disease and ARDS. Moreover, use of elevated positive end-expiratory pressure during mechanical ventilation induces an increase in right ventricular afterload and wall stress, leading to a higher risk of further reducing cardiac output in presence of a failing heart. A major challenge is to distinguish the COVID-19 induced lung damage from *de novo* or coexisting acute cardiogenic pulmonary edema. Historically, right heart catheterization was used to determine pulmonary capillary wedge pressure in order to aid in this distinction, however, this has been omitted from the Berlin criteria for the diagnosis of ARDS. Rather, the Berlin criteria utilize timing of symptom onset, imaging with bilateral pulmonary opacities, and lack of volume overload to identify patients with ARDS. Evaluation by CT chest imaging, lung ultrasound and echocardiography appears to be crucial in this scenario. However, if these diagnostic modalities fails to differentiate and there is still a concern for mixed presentation, pulmonary artery catheterization should be considered in select cases to assess filling pressures, cardiac output and to guide clinical decision-making, given the different management approaches for ARDS and cardiogenic shock. Finally, it is crucial to determine whether or not a concomitant cardiogenic component is present when considering mechanical respiratory and circulatory support with ECMO or other techniques, as this may lend to changes in device selection (venovenous vs veno-arterial ECMO). In a case series of 52 critically ill COVID-19 patients, 83.3% (5/6) of patients who were treated with ECMO did not survive. Further studies are required regarding the utility of ECMO support in advanced COVID-19 cases to clarify which patients may benefit and whether concomitant left ventricular unloading should be done.

Angiotensin Converting Enzyme (ACE) Inhibitors in COVID-19

The SARS-CoV-2 virus enters the cell through binding of spike protein to ACE-2 receptor expressed on the alveolar membrane. ACE-2 predominantly catalyses the conversion of angiotensin II to angiotensin 1-7, and its lesser action is on conversion of angiotensin I to angiotensin 1-9. ACE-2 is present at lung alveolar epithelial cells, heart and kidneys. It is having protective effects on the cardiovascular system by degrading angiotensin II, and acts as a vasodilator. After entry inside the cell, SARS-CoV-2 replicates inside the cell, and cause down regulation of ACE2. The protective role of ACE 2 vanishes and high levels of angiotensin II in the vascular system causes vasoconstriction, acute lung injury and myocardial injury. The authors who had proposed a theoretical hypothesis of an adverse impact of RAAS inhibition in these patients had speculated regarding the upregulation of ACE2 receptors by ACE inhibitors or ARBs in diabetic/hypertensive patients thus helping the entry of virus inside cell. In contrast many other studies showed that ACEi/ARBs are in fact potentiate lung protective function of ACE2, which is an angiotensin II inhibitor. Furthermore, there is a robust evidence of the mortality lowering benefit of ACEi/ARB's in heart failure and postmyocardial infarction. Sudden discontinuation of heart failure therapy leads to precipitation of heart failure. Similarly, ACEi/ARB's, are part of the standard therapy in hypertension, and sudden withdrawal will cause rebound hypertension. Recent literature has firmly emphasized on the need for continuation of these drugs.

Cardiac Arrhythmia

Cardiac arrhythmias including both tachy—as well as bradyarrhythmias are commonly encountered in COVID-19 patients. Our understanding regarding the arrhythmo-genicity in COVID-19 patients is still in nascent phase and is evolving. The etiology of arrhythmias in COVID-19 is often thought to be multifactorial. Arrhythmias may occur due to myocardial damage (myocarditis, ACS, stress cardiomyopathy) or as an indirect manifestation of hypoxic injury, metabolic disarray, myocardial strain, neurohormonal imbalance and adverse effects of drugs. In the initial studies from China, Wang *et al* documented cardiac arrhythmias in 16.7% patients which was frequently being observed in critically ill patients. However, the type and duration of cardiac arrhythmias were not reported. Kunal and colleagues in a series from India reported ECG findings in 108 hospitalized COVID-19 patients. They documented sinus tachycardia in 18 (16.9%), first degree AV block in 5 (4.6%), ventricular tachycardia (VT)/ventricular fibrillation (VF) in 2 (1.8%) and sinus bradycardia in one (0.9%). Tachyarrhythmias frequently encountered in patients with COVID-19 include supraventricular tachycardia (SVT), atrial flutter, atrial fibrillation (AF), monomorphic/ polymorphic VT and VF. Sinus tachycardia is the most common rhythm abnormality among COVID-19 patients and reflects the heightened sympathetic activity during the acute stages of infection. Colon and colleagues evaluated atrial arrhythmias in COVID-19 subsets and reported new-onset atrial tachyarrhythmias including atrial tachycardia, atrial flutter, and AF in 16.5% of hospitalized patients. Guo *et al* in his retrospective case series reported ventricular tachycardia/ventricular fibrillation in 11/187 (5.9%) patients with SARS-CoV-2 infection. They observed that patients with elevated cardiac troponins had a significantly higher frequency of malignant arrhythmias compared to those without (p <0.001). This highlighted the fact that patients with acute myocardial injury and myocarditis had far greater prevalence of tachyarrhythmias. In a global survey by the Heart Rhythm Society among 1197 EP professionals regarding prevalence of arrhythmia in hospitalized COVID-19 patients, AF was the most common tachyarrhythmia while ventricular premature complexes (VPCs) were most commonly reported ventricular arrhythmias (monomorphic VPCs: 5.3%; polymorphic VPCs: 3.5%) followed by NSVT (6.3%). Monomorphic and polymorphic VT was reported by 3.8% and 3.5% respectively and pulseless electrical activity (PEA) by 5.6%. New onset of malignant tachyarrhythmias in the setting of troponin elevation should raise suspicion for underlying myocarditis.

Bradyarrhythmias, such as sinus bradycardia, sinus node dysfunction and complete heart block (CHB) are commonly encountered among patients with COVID-19. In the largest case series of bradyarrhythmia in COVID-19 patients from India, of the seven patients with bradyarrhythmias, five had complete heart block while two had sick sinus syndrome. All the five patients with complete heart block received permanent pacemaker implantation after two weeks of observation for return to sinus rhythm whereas two patients with sinus node dysfunction were kept on close medical follow-up. Only one patient with complete heart block had elevated cardiac troponin marker of myocardial injury thus, the definitive mechanism for the development of bradyarrhythmia in patients with COVID-19 still remains speculative. In another series on severe bradyarrhythmias, authors reported high short-term mortality and morbidity, despite lack of coexistent cardiomyopathy or acute cardiac injury and prompt management of bradycardia with pacing support.

Drug-induced arrhythmias are common in COVID-19 patients. Drug therapies, including hydroxychloroquine (HCQ), chloroquine, lopinavir/ritonavir and azithromycin are known to increase the risk of Torsades de pointes (TdP) due to QT prolongation, especially in critically ill patients with COVID-19. Both chloroquine and HCQ, is structurally similar to quinidine and demonstrates QT-prolonging effects by blocking the activation of potassium channel IKr (hERG/Kv11.1). Also, these drugs are metabolized by cytochrome P450 3A4 (CYP3A4), hence coadministration of other medications that inhibit CYP3A4 enzyme such as statins may result in elevated plasma levels of chloroquine and HCQ. Many drugs in isolation as well as in combination pose a significant risk of QTc prolongation and TdP. In a series of 108 COVID 19 patients from India, among the patients who had received both HCQ and azithromycin therapy had a significant prolongation of QTc (452.5 ± 41.7 ms vs 427.2 ± 22.6 ms; $P = 0.003$) as compared with those who received HCQ alone. Prolongation of QTc was reported in 23.9% of patients who had received both HCQ and azithromycin compared to 3.5% with HCQ alone ($p = 0.009$).

Baseline QTc interval needs to be determined before administration of these drugs. In patients with baseline QTc >500 ms, it is imperative to avoid QT-prolonging drugs. However, at times, it may be reasonable to start therapy with these drugs when the benefits of HCQ is greater than the risk of drug-induced sudden cardiac death. In these patients, QTc should be obtained after 2–4 hours following the first dose and then repeated at 48 hours and 96 hours. In patients with baseline QTc <500 ms, repeat ECG is advocated at 48 or 96 hours following drug initiation. If on therapy QTc is >500 ms or an increase in QTc is >60 ms on serial ECGs monitoring withdrawal of the drug in view of increased risk of TdP and measurements of electrolytes is required. Patients who presents with sustained TdP are usually unstable and may collapse rapidly; they should be resuscitated as per the standard protocols and algorithms of advanced cardiac life support, including cardiac defibrillation. Intravenous magnesium sulfate, anti-tachycardia pacing and intravenous infusion of isoproterenol are useful for managing TdP.

Various cardiological societies have published consensus document for management of arrhythmias in patients with COVID-19. Since these arrhythmias are transient and associated with drug-drug interactions, aggressive management is often not warranted. It must be highlighted that the focus must be on the prevention of cardiac arrhythmias, especially in critically ill patients. Currently, the guidelines do not advocate prophylactic antiarrhythmic agents in patients with COVID-19. In patients with atrial tachyarrhythmias, it is always imperative to identify and treat the secondary causes like hypoxia, metabolic and electrolyte disturbances, and myocardial ischemia. Another important issue regarding the management of AF is the need for anti-coagulation. COVID-19 infection is usually associated with a hypercoagulable state, which increases the risk for subsequent thromboembolism, especially in critically ill patients with markedly elevated D-dimer levels. Thus, prompt anticoagulation is mandated especially where a rhythm control is planned. In patients with brady-arrhythmias, implantation of a temporary pacemaker before permanent pacing can be considered owing to the transient nature of bradyarrhythmias coupled with a greater risk of device infection in these critically ill patients. Assessment should be made regarding the need for a permanent pacemaker post recovery from COVID-19 infection.

Immunothrombosis and Venous Thromboembolism

The clinical course in COVID-19 infection may be complicated by the thrombotic events predominantly venous thromboembolism (VTE). It is associated with increasing disease severity and worse clinical outcomes. Multifactorial processes contributes to VTE and immunothrombosis. Distinctive microvascular abnormalities observed in COVID-19 include endothelial inflammation, disruption of intercellular junctions and microthrombi formation. Patients with COVID-19 can have mild thrombocytopenia, mildly prolonged prothrombin time, increased fibrinogen and raised D-dimer levels, this pattern is known as COVID-19 associated coagulopathy (CAC). It shares pattern with disseminated intravascular coagulation (DIC) but it is a distinct entity. In addition to CAC, critically ill patients often develop venous stasis with prolonged immobilization and are inherently at high-risk for VTE. Hypoxia that occurs in moderate-to-severe COVID-19 illness can lead to endothelial dysfunction and hyper-coagulability. COVID-19-associated coagulopathy along with increased cytokines and activation of platelets, endothelium and complement occur in COVID-19 patients with worsening disease severity. This proinflammatory milieu causes dysregulation of host defence mechanism, leading to excess formation of immunologically mediated thrombi which predominantly affect the microvasculature resulting in immuno-thrombosis.

Occasional cases reported from China and India mentioning occurrence of PE in COVID-19. In a series of 107 consecutive COVID-19 patients from France in critical care setting, 20.6% (22/107) developed pulmonary embolism (PE) as compared to 6.1% COVID-19 negative ICU patients despite having similar severity score (20.6% vs 6.1%; absolute increased risk, 14.4%). Similarly, in an another series of 184 critically ill COVID-19 patients, incidence of composite endpoint of acute PE, deep-vein thrombosis, ischemic stroke, myocardial infarction or systemic arterial embolism was reported to be 31%. This remarkably high incidence of thrombotic events in ICU patients with COVID-19 infections reinforce thrombotic prophylaxis recommendations in critically ill COVID-19 patients. Grillet and colleagues reported incidence of PE to be 23% in severe COVID-19 illness with multivariate analysis showing a higher frequency in males and those on invasive mechanical ventilation. The symptoms and signs of PE are difficult to recognize in the setting of critically ill COVID-19 patients and create a delay in the diagnosis of PE. Acute worsening of hypoxia, hemodynamic instability and unexplained sinus tachycardia should arouse suspicion of PE. D-dimers are usually raised due to the cytokine storm in COVID-19 and will not help in diagnosing PE. Guidelines and position statements from the radiological societies such as European Society of Radiology and the European Society of Thoracic imaging suggest that computed tomography pulmonary angiography (CTPA) to rule out PE should be done if there is need of supplementary oxygen in COVID-19 pneumonia patients with "limited pulmonary involvement."

Controversy exists regarding the use of routine thromboprophylaxis in COVID-19 patients with a few authors supporting the use of low molecular weight heparin in patients with severe pneumonia and excessive activation of coagulation cascade. However, a recent study showed that prophylactic anticoagulation did not avoid the occurrence of PE in hospitalized patients. The CHEST guidelines on prevention, diagnosis and treatment of VTE in COVID-19 advocates for anticoagulant thrombo-prophylaxis in acutely ill hospitalized/critically ill patients. The optimal thromboprophylactic regimen for patients hospitalized with COVID-19 related illness is unknown. Given the drug-drug interactions between some antiviral treatments and direct oral anticoagulants, low molecular weight heparins, or unfractionated heparin with or without mechanical prophylaxis are likely to be preferred in acutely ill hospitalized patients. Management of PE in COVID-19 patients is in line with COVID negative patients. As per the European Society of Cardiology Guidelines, in patients with overt hemodynamic instability (high-risk PE) systemic fibrinolysis is indicated while most of the intermediate-risk hemodynamically stable patients can be managed with anti-coagulation and closely monitored.

Post-COVID-19 CV Sequelae

In the majority of COVID-19 patients, disease course is often uneventful leading to complete recovery from the initial bout of infection. "Post-COVID-19 syndrome" refers to constellation of signs and symptoms in the convalescent phase of the disease process often as a sequelae to the initial COVID-19 infection. Greenhalgh and colleagues defined "post-acute COVID-19" as symptoms that have extended beyond three weeks of the onset of illness and "chronic COVID-19" as symptoms extending beyond 12 weeks of onset of illness. Various published studies reported "post COVID-19 syndrome" in a range of 30–87.4% of patients recovered from COVID-19. The spectrum of post COVID-19 cardiovascular sequelae comprises of ACS, myocarditis, pericarditis, cardiac arrhythmias, thromboembolic events especially VTE and cardiac autonomic dysfunction. Clinical symptoms of post-COVID-19 cardiovascular sequelae includes chest pain, palpitation, dyspnea, presyncope and syncope. Mechanisms perpetuating cardiovascular sequelae in post-COVID-19 syndrome include direct viral invasion, downregulation of ACE2, inflammation, hypercoagulable state and the immunologic response affecting the structural integrity of the myocardium, pericardium and conduction system. Autonomic dysfunction after viral illness, resulting in postural orthostatic tachycardia syndrome and inappropriate sinus tachycardia results from adrenergic modulation.

Serial clinical and imaging evaluation with electrocardiogram and echocardiogram at 4–12 weeks may be considered in those with cardiovascular complications during acute infection, or persistent cardiac symptoms. Current evidence does not support the routine utilization of advanced cardiac imaging, and this should be considered on a case-by-case basis. Patients with post-COVID-19 ACS should be treated as per standard protocol. They should be continued on postmyocardial infarction (MI) therapies including ACE inhibitors and/or beta-blockers along with serial imaging follow-up for ventricular functions. Conclusive evidence is not yet available for extended post-hospital discharge (up to 6 weeks) and prolonged primary thromboprophylaxis (up to 45 day) in those managed as outpatients. It may have a more favorable risk-benefit ratio in COVID-19 patients given the increase risk of thrombotic complications during the acute and convalescent phase, and this is still an area of active investigation. The CHEST guidelines on VTE prevention in COVID-19 recommends only inpatient anticoagulant thromboprophylaxis over inpatient plus extended thromboprophylaxis after hospital discharge. Elevated D-dimer levels, in addition to comorbidities such as cancer and immobility, may help to risk stratify patients at the highest risk of postacute thrombosis; however, individual patient-level considerations for risk versus benefit should dictate recommendations at this time. Direct oral anticoagulants and low-molecular-weight heparin are preferred anticoagulation agents over vitamin K antagonists due to the lack of need to frequently monitor therapeutic levels, as well as the lower risk of drug–drug interactions. Therapeutic anticoagulation for those with imaging-confirmed VTE is recommended for ≥3 months, similar to provoked VTE. The role of antiplatelet agents such as aspirin as an alternative or in conjunction with anticoagulation agents for thromboprophylaxis in COVID-19 has not yet been defined and is currently being investigated as a prolonged primary thromboprophylaxis strategy in those managed as outpatients. Physical activity and ambulation should be recommended to all patients when appropriate. Patients with postural orthostatic tachycardia syndrome and inappropriate sinus tachycardia may benefit from a low-dose beta blocker for heart rate management and reducing adrenergic activity.

Catheterization Lab Considerations During COVID-19 Pandemic

The American as well as European CV association position statements proposed that elective procedures should be abandoned in the catheterization laboratory. The rationale was to reduce the number of elective hospitalizations to increase bed capacity for COVID-19 patients; to reduce exposure of individuals (i.e. patients and their relatives) to high-risk hospital environment; and to reduce the exposure of Health care workers (HCWs) to asymptomatic COVID-19 patients. However, it is imperative to take a case by case individualized decision taking into account the risk of COVID-19 exposure versus the risk of delaying the diagnosis or treatment should be done. EAPCI position statement have categorized invasive procedure based on the urgency of treatment as illustrated in Table 16.3. Emergency cardiac procedures should be performed, after wearing personal protective equipment (PPE) including gown, gloves, goggles or shields, and a N95 mask. The catheterization labs should be equipped with powered air purifying respirator (PAPR) systems, especially for patients who may require cardiopulmonary resuscitation (CPR) and/or intubation. Of note vast majority of catheterization labs have either normal or positive ventilation systems and are not

TABLE 16.3: Categorizing invasive procedure during COVID-19 pandemic

Emergent (do not postpone)	Urgent (perform within days)	Lower priority (perform within <3 months)	Elective (may be postponed >3 months)
1. STEMI 2. Very high-risk and high-risk NSTE-ACS 3. Cardiogenic shock	1. Intermediate risk NSTE-ACS 2. Unstable angina 3. Left main PCI 4. Last remaining vessel PCI 5. Decompensated ischemic heart failure 6. Angina pectoris class IV 7. CABG in patients with NSTE-ACS unsuitable for PCI 8. Urgent heart transplant	1. Advanced CAD with angina class III or NYHA III symptoms 2. Staged PCI of non-IRA in STEMI in patients with hemodynamic stability and without >90% lesions in proximal segments of major epicardial coronary arteries 3. Proximal LAD PCI 4. LVAD	1. CTO interventions 2. CCS with angina class II or NYHA II symptoms

designed for infection isolation. Therefore, catheterization labs will require a thorough cleaning and disinfection following the procedure leading to delays for subsequent procedures. If possible for COVID-19 positive patients, restriction of cases to a dedicated laboratory will make it helpful.

Life saving measure like endotracheal intubation, suctioning, bag and mask ventilation and CPR results in aerosol generation increasing likelihood of exposure to healthcare personnel. In the event of a cardiac arrest, one measure which may help protect healthcare workers is the use of external mechanical compression devices to minimize direct contact with infected patients. Patients who are already intubated pose less of a transmission risk because their ventilation is managed through a closed circuit. Patients with COVID-19 or suspected COVID-19 requiring intubation should be intubated prior to arrival to the catheterization laboratory. Further, the threshold to consider intubation in a patient with borderline respiratory status may need to be lowered in order to avoid emergent intubation in the catheterization laboratory. Use a HEPA (high efficiency particulate air) filter between the tubes and bag if bag ventilation is being done to decrease aerosolization. Other considerations is to use closed circuit BIPAP/CPAP (bilevel or continuous positive airway pressure) machines if intubation not available. Close coordination with critical care and cardiac anesthesia teams in airway management will be critical to avoid spread of infection.

Down sizing case volumes and shift-based allocation of physicians, paramedical staff, and technician to operate the lab without disruption. Procedures which can be performed bedside should be performed thereto to prevent risk to contracting infection during transportation from ward to laboratory. In addition to avoid shortage of N95 masks and PPE there should be reduction in the number of people being scrub into procedures.

Triaging CV Patients and Follow-up Visits

Telemedicine can help in prevention of transmission of virus and is ideal in this public health crises. It allows triage of patients while minimizing exposure of patients and healthcare professional to potential infection. Additionally, it provides an opportunity for specialists that might otherwise not available to evaluate patients. There is a need to minimize non-essential/non-urgent in-person provider–patient interactions as much as possible.

CONCLUSIONS AND FUTURE DIRECTIONS

COVID-19 pandemic has affected hundreds of thousands of Indians during this second wave and have posed a major challenge in terms of public health. CV comorbidities are common in patients with COVID-19 and such patients are at heightened risk of morbidity and mortality. Apart from respiratory failure, SARS CoV-2 infection causes a wide spectrum of CV manifestation both during acute phase and post recovery and are associated with worse prognosis. CV community will play a key role in management of patients affected by COVID-19. CV society will need to come up with guidelines for management of CVD patients with and without COVD-19 simultaneously without compromising safety. In the coming time every efforts should be made to vaccinate the community to prevent rapid spread of infection. It will be crucial to develop newer therapies to overcome this multisystem viral disease. In addition, prospective randomized trials and cohort studies should be conducted to further standardize treatment of these patients. Various stakeholders should come together and make healthcare system more efficient to improve outcomes of these patients.

BIBLIOGRAPHY

1. Adeghate EA, Eid N, Singh J. Mechanisms of COVID-19-induced heart failure: a short review. Heart Fail Rev. 2021 Mar;26(2):363–9.

2. Agstam S, Vijay J, Gupta A, Bansal S. Acute pulmonary embolism: An unseen villain in COVID-19. Indian Heart J. 2020 May-Jun;72(3):218–9.

3. Barnes GD, Burnett A, Allen A, Blumenstein M, Clark NP, Cuker A, et al. Thromboembolism and anticoagulant therapy during the COVID-19 pandemic: interim clinical guidance from the anticoagulation forum. J Thromb Thrombolysis. 2020 Jul;50(1):72–81.

4. Bompard F, Monnier H, Saab I, Tordjman M, Abdoul H, Fournier L, et al. Pulmonary embolism in patients with COVID-19 pneumonia. Eur Respir J. 2020 Jul 30;56(1):2001365.

5. Cameli M, Pastore MC, Mandoli GE, D'Ascenzi F, Focardi M, Biagioni G, et al. COVID-19 and Acute Coronary Syndromes: Current Data and Future Implications. Front Cardiovasc Med. 2021 Jan 28;7:593496.

6. Carfi A, Bernabei R, Landi F; Gemelli Against COVID-19 Post-Acute Care Study Group. Persistent Symptoms in Patients After Acute COVID-19. JAMA. 2020 Aug 11;324(6):603–5. doi: 10.1001/jama.2020.12603.

7. Chieffo A, Stefanini GG, Price S, Barbato E, Tarantini G, Karam N, et al. EAPCI Position Statement on Invasive Management of Acute Coronary Syndromes during the COVID-19 pandemic. Eur Heart J. 2020 May 14;41(19):1839–51.

8. Chinitz JS, Goyal R, Harding M, Veseli G, Gruberg L, Jadonath R, et al. Bradyarrhythmias in patients with COVID-19: Marker of poor prognosis? Pacing Clin Electrophysiol. 2020 Oct;43(10):1199–1204.

9. Colon CM, Barrios JG, Chiles JW, McElwee SK, Russell DW, Maddox WR, et al. Atrial Arrhythmias in COVID-19 Patients. JACC Clin Electrophysiol. 2020 Sep;6(9):1189–90.

10. Cucinotta D, Vanelli M. WHO Declares COVID-19 a Pandemic. Acta Biomed. 2020 Mar 19;91(1):157–60.

11. Danzi GB, Loffi M, Galeazzi G, Gherbesi E. Acute pulmonary embolism and COVID-19 pneumonia: a random association? Eur Heart J. 2020 May 14;41(19):1858.

12. Dherange P, Lang J, Qian P, Oberfeld B, Sauer WH, Koplan B, et al. Arrhythmias and COVID-19: A Review. JACC Clin Electrophysiol. 2020 Sep;6(9):1193–1204.

13. Fang L, Karakiulakis G, Roth M. Are patients with hypertension and diabetes mellitus at increased risk for COVID-19 infection? Lancet Respir Med. 2020 Apr;8(4):e21.

14. Ferguson ND, Fan E, Camporota L, Antonelli M, Anzueto A, Beale R, et al. The Berlin definition of ARDS: an expanded rationale, justification, and supplementary material. Intensive Care Med. 2012 Oct;38(10):1573–82.

15. Ferrario CM, Jessup J, Chappell MC, Averill DB, Brosnihan KB, Tallant EA, et al. Effect of angiotensin-converting enzyme inhibition and angiotensin II receptor blockers on cardiac angiotensin-converting enzyme 2. Circulation. 2005 May 24;111(20):2605–10.

16. Goldstein DS. The possible association between COVID-19 and postural tachycardia syndrome. Heart Rhythm. 2021 Apr;18(4):508–9.

17. Gopinathannair R, Merchant FM, Lakkireddy DR, Etheridge SP, Feigofsky S, Han JK, et al. COVID-19 and cardiac arrhythmias: a global perspective on arrhythmia characteristics and management strategies. J Interv Card Electrophysiol. 2020 Nov; 59(2):329–36.

18. Greenhalgh T, Knight M, A'Court C, Buxton M, Husain L. Management of post-acute covid-19 in primary care. BMJ. 2020 Aug 11;370:m3026.

19. Grillet F, Behr J, Calame P, Aubry S, Delabrousse E. Acute Pulmonary Embolism Associated with COVID-19 Pneumonia Detected with Pulmonary CT Angiography. Radiology. 2020 Sep;296(3):E186–8.

20. Guan WJ, Ni ZY, Hu Y, Liang WH, Ou CQ, He JX, et al. China Medical Treatment Expert Group for Covid-19. Clinical Characteristics of Coronavirus Disease 2019 in China. N Engl J Med. 2020 Apr 30;382(18):1708–20.

21. Guo T, Fan Y, Chen M, Wu X, Zhang L, He T, et al. Cardiovascular Implications of Fatal Outcomes of Patients With Coronavirus Disease 2019 (COVID-19). JAMA Cardiol. 2020 Jul 1;5(7):811–8.

22. Guo YR, Cao QD, Hong ZS, Tan YY, Chen SD, Jin HJ, et al. The origin, transmission and clinical therapies on coronavirus disease 2019 (COVID-19) outbreak—an update on the status. Mil Med Res. 2020 Mar 13;7(1):11.

23. Gupta MD, Qamar A, Mp G, Safal S, Batra V, Basia D, et al. Bradyarrhythmias in patients with COVID-19: A case series. Indian Pacing Electrophysiol J. 2020 Sep-Oct;20(5):211–2.

24. Gupta N, Zhao YY, Evans CE. The stimulation of thrombosis by hypoxia. Thromb Res. 2019 Sep;181:77–83.

25. Hoffmann M, Kleine-Weber H, Schroeder S, Krüger N, Herrler T, Erichsen S, et al. SARS-CoV-2 Cell Entry Depends on ACE2 and TMPRSS2 and Is Blocked by a Clinically Proven Protease Inhibitor. Cell. 2020 Apr 16;181(2):271–80.e8.

26. Hu H, Ma F, Wei X, Fang Y. Coronavirus fulminant myocarditis treated with glucocorticoid and human immunoglobulin. Eur Heart J. 2021 Jan 7;42(2):206.

27. Huang C, Huang L, Wang Y, Li X, Ren L, Gu X, et al. 6-month consequences of COVID-19 in patients discharged from hospital: a cohort study. Lancet. 2021 Jan 16;397(10270):220–32.

28. Iba T, Levy JH, Connors JM, Warkentin TE, Thachil J, Levi M. The unique characteristics of COVID-19 coagulopathy. Crit Care. 2020 Jun 18;24(1):360.

29. Imai Y, Kuba K, Rao S, Huan Y, Guo F, Guan B, et al. Angiotensin-converting enzyme 2 protects from severe acute lung failure. Nature. 2005 Jul 7;436(7047):112–6.

30. Jing ZC, Zhu HD, Yan XW, Chai WZ, Zhang S. Recommendations from the Peking Union Medical College Hospital for the management of acute myocardial infarction during the COVID-19 outbreak. Eur Heart J. 2020 May 14;41(19):1791–4.

31. Kang Y, Chen T, Mui D, Ferrari V, Jagasia D, Scherrer-Crosbie M, et al. Cardiovascular manifestations and treatment considerations in COVID-19. Heart. 2020 Aug;106(15):1132–41.

32. Klok FA, Kruip MJHA, van der Meer NJM, Arbous MS, Gommers DAMPJ, Kant KM, et al. Incidence of thrombotic complications in critically ill ICU patients with COVID-19. Thromb Res. 2020 Jul;191:145–7.

33. Konstantinides SV, Meyer G, Becattini C, Bueno H, Geersing GJ, Harjola VP, et al. ESC Scientific Document Group. 2019 ESC Guidelines for the diagnosis and management of acute pulmonary embolism developed in collaboration with the European Respiratory Society (ERS). Eur Heart J. 2020 Jan 21;41(4):543–603.

34. Kunal S, Gupta K, Sharma SM, Pathak V, Mittal S, Tarke C. Cardiovascular system and COVID-19: perspectives from a developing country. Monaldi Arch Chest Dis. 2020 May 7;90(2).

35. Kunal S, Sharma SM, Sharma SK, Gautam D, Bhatia H, Mahla H, et al. Cardiovascular complications and its impact on outcomes in COVID-19. Indian Heart J. 2020 Nov-Dec;72(6):593–8.

36. Kuster GM, Pfister O, Burkard T, Zhou Q, Twerenbold R, Haaf P, et al. SARS-CoV2: should inhibitors of the renin-angiotensin system be withdrawn in patients with COVID-19? Eur Heart J. 2020 May 14;41(19):1801–3.

37. Lakkireddy DR, Chung MK, Gopinathannair R, Patton KK, Gluckman TJ, Turagam M, et al. Guidance for Cardiac Electrophysiology During the COVID-19 Pandemic from the Heart Rhythm Society COVID-19 Task Force; Electrophysiology Section of the American College of Cardiology; and the Electrocardiography and Arrhythmias Committee of the Council on Clinical Cardiology, American Heart Association. Circulation. 2020 May 26;141(21):e823–31.

38. Lauer SA, Grantz KH, Bi Q, Jones FK, Zheng Q, Meredith HR, et al. The Incubation Period of Coronavirus Disease 2019 (COVID-19) From Publicly Reported Confirmed Cases: Estimation and Application. Ann Intern Med. 2020 May 5;172(9):577–82.

39. Li B, Yang J, Zhao F, Zhi L, Wang X, Liu L, et al. Prevalence and impact of cardiovascular metabolic diseases on COVID-19 in China. Clin Res Cardiol. 2020 May;109(5):531–8.

40. Loo J, Spittle DA, Newnham M. COVID-19, immunothrombosis and venous thromboembolism: biological mechanisms. Thorax. 2021 Jan 6:thoraxjnl-2020-216243. doi: 10.1136/thoraxjnl-2020-216243. Epub ahead of print.

41. MacLaren G, Fisher D, Brodie D. Preparing for the Most Critically Ill Patients With COVID-19: The Potential Role of Extracorporeal Membrane Oxygenation. JAMA. 2020 Apr 7;323(13):1245–6.

42. Moores LK, Tritschler T, Brosnahan S, Carrier M, Collen JF, Doerschug K, et al. Prevention, Diagnosis, and Treatment of VTE in Patients With Coronavirus Disease 2019: CHEST Guideline and Expert Panel Report. Chest. 2020 Sep;158(3):1143–63.

43. Nahum J, Morichau-Beauchant T, Daviaud F, Echegut P, Fichet J, Maillet JM, et al. Venous Thrombosis Among Critically Ill Patients With Coronavirus Disease 2019 (COVID-19). JAMA Netw Open. 2020 May 1;3(5):e2010478.

44. Nalbandian A, Sehgal K, Gupta A, Madhavan MV, McGroder C, Stevens JS, et al. Post-acute COVID-19 syndrome. Nat Med. 2021 Apr;27(4):601–15.

45. Nishiga M, Wang DW, Han Y, Lewis DB, Wu JC. COVID-19 and cardiovascular disease: from basic mechanisms to clinical perspectives. Nat Rev Cardiol. 2020 Sep;17(9):543–58.

46. Perrin R, Riste L, Hann M, Walther A, Mukherjee A, Heald A. Into the looking glass: Post-viral syndrome post COVID-19. Med Hypotheses. 2020 Nov;144:110055.

47. Poissy J, Goutay J, Caplan M, Parmentier E, Duburcq T, Lassalle F, et al. Lille ICU Haemostasis COVID-19 Group. Pulmonary Embolism in Patients With COVID-19: Awareness of an Increased Prevalence. Circulation. 2020 Jul 14;142(2):184–6.

48. Puntmann VO, Carerj ML, Wieters I, Fahim M, Arendt C, Hoffmann J, et al. Outcomes of Cardiovascular Magnetic Resonance Imaging in Patients Recently Recovered From Coronavirus Disease 2019 (COVID-19). JAMA Cardiol. 2020 Nov 1;5(11):1265–73.

49. Raj SR, Black BK, Biaggioni I, Paranjape SY, Ramirez M, Dupont WD, et al. Propranolol decreases tachycardia and improves symptoms in the postural tachycardia syndrome: less is more. Circulation. 2009 Sep 1;120(9):725–34.

50. Ramakrishnan S, Jabir A, Jayagopal PB, Mohanan PP, Nair VK, Das MK, et al. Pattern of acute MI admissions in India during COVID-19 era: A Cardiological Society of India study - Rationale and design. Indian Heart J. 2020 Nov-Dec;72(6):541–6.

51. Revel MP, Parkar AP, Prosch H, Silva M, Sverzellati N, Gleeson F, et al. European Society of Radiology (ESR) and the European Society of Thoracic Imaging (ESTI). COVID-19 patients and the radiology department–advice from the European Society of Radiology (ESR) and the European Society of Thoracic Imaging (ESTI). Eur Radiol. 2020 Sep;30(9):4903–9.

52. Ruan Q, Yang K, Wang W, Jiang L, Song J. Clinical predictors of mortality due to COVID-19 based on an analysis of data of 150 patients from Wuhan, China. Intensive Care Med. 2020 May;46(5):846–8.

53. Saenz LC, Miranda A, Speranza R, Texeira RA, Rojel U, Enriquez A, et al. Recommendations for the organization of electrophysiology and cardiac pacing services during the COVID-19 pandemic : Latin American Heart Rhythm Society (LAHRS) in collaboration with: Colombian College Of Electrophysiology, Argentinian Society of Cardiac Electrophysiology (SADEC), Brazilian Society Of Cardiac Arrhythmias (SOBRAC), Mexican Society Of Cardiac Electrophysiology (SOMEEC). J Interv Card Electrophysiol. 2020 Nov;59(2):307–13.

54. Shi S, Qin M, Shen B, Cai Y, Liu T, Yang F, et al. Association of Cardiac Injury With Mortality in Hospitalized Patients With COVID-19 in Wuhan, China. JAMA Cardiol. 2020 Jul 1;5(7):802–10.

55. Showkathali R, Yalamanchi R, Sankeerthana MP, Kumaran SN, Shree S, Nayak R, et al. Acute Coronary Syndrome admissions and outcome during COVID-19 Pandemic-Report from large tertiary centre in India. Indian Heart J. 2020 Nov-Dec;72(6):599–602.

56. Sisti N, Valente S, Mandoli GE, Santoro C, Sciaccaluga C, Franchi F, et al. COVID-19 in patients with heart failure: the new and the old epidemic. Postgrad Med J. 2021 Mar;97(1145): 175–9.

57. Starekova J, Bluemke DA, Bradham WS, Eckhardt LL, Grist TM, Kusmirek JE, et al. Evaluation for Myocarditis in Competitive Student Athletes Recovering From Coronavirus Disease 2019 With Cardiac Magnetic Resonance Imaging. JAMA Cardiol. 2021 Jan 14:e207444.

58. Su S, Wong G, Shi W, Liu J, Lai ACK, Zhou J, et al. Epidemiology, Genetic Recombination, and Pathogenesis of Coronaviruses. Trends Microbiol. 2016 Jun;24(6):490–502.

59. Tam CF, Cheung KS, Lam S, Wong A, Yung A, Sze M, et al. Impact of Coronavirus Disease 2019 (COVID-19) Outbreak on ST-Segment-Elevation Myocardial Infarction Care in Hong Kong, China. Circ Cardiovasc Qual Outcomes. 2020 Apr;13(4):e006631.

60. Thomas SH, Behr ER. Pharmacological treatment of acquired QT prolongation and torsades de pointes. Br J Clin Pharmacol. 2016 Mar;81(3):420–7.

61. Vaduganathan M, Vardeny O, Michel T, McMurray JJV, Pfeffer MA, Solomon SD. Renin-Angiotensin-Aldosterone System Inhibitors in Patients with Covid-19. N Engl J Med. 2020 Apr 23;382(17):1653–9.

62. Wang D, Hu B, Hu C, Zhu F, Liu X, Zhang J, et al. Clinical Characteristics of 138 Hospitalized Patients With 2019 Novel Coronavirus-Infected Pneumonia in Wuhan, China. JAMA. 2020 Mar 17;323(11):1061–9.

63. Wang H, Yang P, Liu K, Guo F, Zhang Y, Zhang G, et al. SARS coronavirus entry into host cells through a novel clathrin- and caveolae-independent endocytic pathway. Cell Res. 2008 Feb;18(2):290–301.

64. Welt FGP, Shah PB, Aronow HD, Bortnick AE, Henry TD, Sherwood MW, et al. American College of Cardiology's Interventional Council and the Society for Cardiovascular Angiography and Interventions. Catheterization Laboratory Considerations During the Coronavirus (COVID-19) Pandemic: From the ACC's Interventional Council and SCAI. J Am Coll Cardiol. 2020 May 12;75(18):2372–5.

65. WHO. Coronavirus disease. Accessed on: 29 May 2021. Available from: https://covid19.who.int/region/searo/country/in

66. Wu D, Wu T, Liu Q, Yang Z. The SARS-CoV-2 outbreak: What we know. Int J Infect Dis. 2020 May;94:44–8.

67. Wu Z, McGoogan JM. Characteristics of and Important Lessons From the Coronavirus Disease 2019 (COVID-19) Outbreak in China: Summary of a Report of 72/314 Cases From the Chinese Center for Disease Control and Prevention. JAMA. 2020 Apr 7;323(13):1239–42.

68. Xie Y, Wang X, Yang P, Zhang S. COVID-19 Complicated by Acute Pulmonary Embolism. Radiol Cardiothorac Imaging. 2020 Mar 16;2(2):e200067.

69. Yang J, Zheng Y, Gou X, Pu K, Chen Z, Guo Q, et al. Prevalence of comorbidities and its effects in patients infected with SARS-CoV-2: a systematic review and meta-analysis. Int J Infect Dis. 2020 May;94:91–5.

70. Zeng JH, Liu YX, Yuan J, Wang FX, Wu WB, Li JX, et al. First case of COVID-19 complicated with fulminant myocarditis: a case report and insights. Infection. 2020 Oct;48(5):773–7.

71. Zhang T, Wu Q, Zhang Z. Probable Pangolin Origin of SARS-CoV-2 Associated with the COVID-19 Outbreak. Curr Biol. 2020 Apr 6;30(7):1346–51.e2.

72. Zhou F, Yu T, Du R, Fan G, Liu Y, Liu Z, et al. Clinical course and risk factors for mortality of adult inpatients with COVID-19 in Wuhan, China: a retrospective cohort study. Lancet. 2020 Mar 28;395(10229):1054–62.

73. Zhu N, Zhang D, Wang W, Li X, Yang B, Song J, et al. China Novel Coronavirus Investigating and Research Team. A Novel Coronavirus from Patients with Pneumonia in China, 2019. N Engl J Med. 2020 Feb 20;382(8):727–33.

Changes in the Clinical Profile and Management of COVID-19 in the Second Wave of the Pandemic

Sandeep Garg, Sricharan V, Sunita Aggarwal

INTRODUCTION

In December 2019, a novel-disease caused by the severe acute respiratory syndrome coronavirus (SARS-CoV-2) was discovered which spread worldwide within a few months. The WHO declared it as a pandemic on 11th March 2020. As of July 2021, more than 180 million infected cases and 4 million deaths have been reported. In most countries, the scenario has been marked by two 'waves' of the pandemic which refers to the cases clustered around a period of time. The first wave of the pandemic in India lasted throughout 2020 and the second wave began in 2021 which peaked during April-May 2021. These waves differed in many aspects including the preparedness and availability of healthcare infrastructure, knowledge and research about the disease, transmissibility, variants of the virus, diagnostic methods, clinical presentations, treatment strategies and preventive measures.

CLINICAL FEATURES AND PRESENTATION

Several studies have shown that the first and second waves of the COVID-19 pandemic in many countries differed in terms of the symptoms at presentation. The most common clinical presentation seen during the first wave was fever, dry cough, fatigue, loss of taste or smell, difficulty in breathing whereas atypical symptoms, such as diarrhea, skin rashes, conjunctivitis, vomiting were reported in the second wave. There was also a difference in the age range of patients affected in both waves as the infections in the second wave encompassed a broad age range from infants and children to older adults. In addition, there was an increase in the number of pregnant women afflicted. The successive waves of the pandemic have witnessed diverse trends in various parts of the world. The factors responsible for the occurrence of the second wave are unclear but the rise in the B.1.617.2 (delta) variant due to its increased transmissibility has been postulated as one of the reasons compared to the dominance of the B.1.1.7 (alpha) variant during the first wave.

In India, the National Clinical Registry for COVID-19 has documented the changes during the second wave of the pandemic compared to the first wave. Compared to the first wave, there was an increase in the following:
- Proportion of cases in the age group of <40 years
- Number of asymptomatic cases

- Proportion of patients presenting with shortness of breath
- Complications such as ARDS and septic shock
- Use of supplemental oxygen and requirement of mechanical ventilation
- Overall mortality rate and across all age groups except <20 years of age
- Number of cases due to mutant strains (B.1.1.7 and B.1.617)

However, a decrease was observed in the proportion of affected males and people with comorbidities. Besides this, another study conducted across a network of hospitals in north India reported the following findings:

- Proportion of severe COVID-19 cases increased
- Mean length of hospital stay decreased
- Increased incidence of secondary bacterial and fungal infections such as UTI, HAP and especially mucormycosis.

COVID-19 associated mucormycosis (CAM) refers to the opportunistic infection by mucormycetes and related fungi in a patient infected with or recovered from COVID-19. The incidence of CAM has surged across the world especially in India, as evidenced by the 2-fold rise in the incidence of mucormycosis during the COVID-19 pandemic. Although the exact incidence of mucormycosis during the first wave is unknown, reports suggest that there has been a phenomenal rise during the second wave. The presence of uncontrolled diabetes and use of corticosteroids appear to be the most important factors for its predisposition.

SARS-COV-2 VARIANTS

Towards the end of 2020, new variants of SARS-CoV-2 began to emerge throughout the world due to mutations in the spike protein leading to differences in the severity of illness, transmissibility and vaccine efficacy. These variants were classified by the PANGO nomenclature and the WHO based on the type of mutations and the place of first reporting. A variant was designated as a variant of concern (VOC) if it displayed increased transmissibility, virulence or had an impact on the diagnosis or the efficacy of treatments or vaccines. The important VOC in circulation at present are as follows:

Variant name (WHO name)	Pango lineage	Mutations of interest	Place and month of first reporting
Alpha	B.1.1.7	N501Y, D614G, P681H	UK, September 2020
Beta	B.1.351	K417N, E484K, N501Y, D614G, A701V	South Africa, September 2020
Gamma	P.1	K417T, E484K, N501Y, D614G, H655Y	Brazil, December 2020
Delta	B.1.617.2	L452R, T478K, D614G, P681R	India, December 2020

CHANGES IN THE MANAGEMENT OF COVID-19

The initial phase of the COVID-19 pandemic in early 2020 created a huge burden on the healthcare system due to limited knowledge about the disease transmission and treatment options. However, the successive months witnessed an array of advancements in the diagnostic and therapeutic modalities for combating COVID-19.

There were many drugs used in both the waves as the data regarding their benefits was available since the early part of the first wave. However, further research led to changes in their use.

Drugs and Therapies Used in both the Waves of the Pandemic

- **Chloroquine, hydroxychloroquine:** These are antimalarials with broad-spectrum antiviral activity which act by inhibition of virus-host cell fusion and viral entry besides suppressing the production of pro-inflammatory cytokines. These were one of the first drugs tested against SARS-CoV-2. Initial studies revealed that these drugs might be useful in the prevention of cytokine storm and hence HCQ was empirically used for treatment and prophylaxis of contacts. But the lack of solid data on mortality benefit and the incidence of serious adverse effects such as arrhythmias, QTc prolongation, retinopathy led to the discontinuation of their use and these drugs were scarcely used in the second wave.
- **Azithromycin and ivermectin:** Azithromycin is an immunomodulatory antibiotic used for the empirical treatment of community-acquired pneumonia. Some studies reported that the combination of HCQ and azithromycin had a synergistic effect on decreasing the SARS-CoV-2 viral load. But the additive adverse effect of QTc prolongation discouraged the use of this combination. Ivermectin, an antiparasitic drug was shown to inhibit viral replication *in vitro*. There has been no conclusive evidence in clinical trials though.
- **Remdesivir:** It is an RNA-dependent RNA polymerase inhibitor originally devised for the treatment of Ebolavirus infection. Initial clinical trials showed that it was effective against SARS-CoV-2. Based on this, the FDA issued emergency use authorization in May 2020. The recovery trial concluded that remdesivir reduces the length of hospital stay and oxygen requirement in moderate and severe patients with COVID-19. The solidarity trial showed that remdesivir failed to demonstrate any mortality benefit along with lopinavir-ritonavir, interferon β and hydroxy-chloroquine. The use of remdesivir in India started in June 2020 and continued throughout the first wave. However, the second wave saw much higher usage comparatively even to an extent that many hospitals and pharmacies ran out of supply.
- **Corticosteroids:** The well-known anti-inflammatory effects of corticosteroids prompted their use in COVID-19 and it was shown that steroids reduced mortality in COVID-19 patients on oxygen support. The recovery trial reinforced this fact by proving that dexamethasone use was associated with decreased mortality in patients receiving oxygen and those on mechanical ventilation. Consequent to this, the usage of steroids in India grew in the first wave and continued with the same intensity in the second wave although dexamethasone was more widely used in the second wave compared to other steroids.
- **Anticoagulants:** The pathogenesis of COVID-19 involves endothelial injury which promotes thrombosis and inflammation, especially in the lung vasculature. Hence the use of anticoagulants such as unfractionated heparin and LMWH in prophylactic dose was advocated in hospitalized COVID-19 patients. There was no significant change in the rate of anticoagulant use between the first and second waves in India.

- **Tocilizumab:** It is a monoclonal antibody which prevents the binding of IL-6 to IL-6 receptors thereby suppressing the action of IL-6 in the cytokine storm. Initial studies showed conflicting results but later studies have shown that tocilizumab decreases mortality and the requirement of mechanical ventilation among severe and critically ill COVID-19 patients. The recovery and the REMAP-CAP trials suggested improved outcomes including survival with tocilizumab in critical COVID-19. In India, tocilizumab was used in both the waves of the pandemic but the extent of difference in usage remains unclear as two studies have yielded conflicting results.
- **Convalescent plasma therapy (CPT):** It is a mode of passive immunization against COVID-19 and involves the administration of plasma from an individual who recently recovered from COVID-19 to the patient. The main mechanism of protection is by the presence of neutralizing antibodies to SARS-CoV-2 proteins. The PLACID trial conducted in India failed to show any benefit in terms of prevention of deterioration or mortality in moderately ill COVID-19 patients. This might probably be due to the low titers of neutralizing antibodies (median 1:40) present in the donor plasma samples. The DCGI has approved the use of CPT as an 'off-label' experimental therapy. The use of CPT in India during both the waves has been almost similar, although it appears to be on a declining trend.

Newer Therapies and Advances seen during the Second Wave of COVID-19

- **Monoclonal antibodies:** Bamlanivimab, etesevimab, casirivimab and imdevimab are monoclonal antibodies that target the spike protein of SARS-CoV-2. After achieving satisfactory results in clinical trials, the FDA and the CDSCO provided EUA for the combination of casirivimab-imdevimab and bamlanivimab-etesivimab for the treatment of COVID-19 patients not on oxygen support and at risk of progression to severe disease.
- **Baricitinib:** It is a JAK-STAT inhibitor originally used for the treatment of rheumatoid arthritis. ACTT-2 trial evaluated the efficacy of combination of remdesivir with baricitinib and found that it was associated with shorter recovery times and higher odds of clinical improvement in those on noninvasive ventilation. The CDSCO later issued EUA for baricitinib in India in May 2021.
- **2-Deoxy-D-glucose:** It is an antimetabolite of glucose which inhibits glycolysis on accumulating in the virus infected cells and thus reduces lung damage and inflammation. 2-DG was jointly developed in India by the INMAS, DRDO and Dr Reddy's labs and was granted EUA by the DCGI in May 2021 after phase-III trial results across many states showed the 2-DG significantly reduced oxygen dependence in moderate and severe COVID-19 patients.

Vaccination in the Second Wave of COVID-19

A major difference between the two waves of the pandemic in India is that the second wave occurred after the beginning of the vaccination against COVID-19. The vaccination program commenced on 16th January 2021 and till date 37 crore doses have been administered of which 7 crore people have received more than one dose.

- **Covishield (ChAdOx-1 nCoV-19 vaccine):** It was developed by AstraZeneca in collaboration with Oxford University, UK and was manufactured by Serum Institute of India, Pune. It consists of the SARS-CoV-2 spike protein incorporated in a chimpanzee adenoviral vector which generates antibodies against the spike protein. The efficacy is reported to be 70% after two doses. The breakthrough infection rate after two doses of Covishield has been reported to be 1.6% and the efficacy of Covishield against the delta variant is reported to be 59.8% according to one study.

- **Covaxin (BBV152 vaccine):** It was developed by Bharat Biotech in collaboration with the ICMR and NIV. It is an inactivated whole virus vaccine which stimulates antibody response against spike protein and other SARS-CoV-2 antigens. It has been reported to show an efficacy of 77.8% against symptomatic COVID-19 and 65.8% against the delta variant according to the results of a phase 3 trial.

CONCLUSION

The second wave of COVID-19 has resulted in significant mortality and morbidity besides posing a huge burden on healthcare resources. Since only a miniscule proportion of the population worldwide is vaccinated, the threat of another wave looms large. An understanding of the SARS-CoV-2 viral dynamics and mutations is necessary to predict future 'waves' and control the pandemic as well as to devise effective treatment and prevention strategies. It is therefore imperative to encourage active research in these fields to be ready to combat the next wave.

BIBLIOGRAPHY

1. Agarwal A, Mukherjee A, Kumar G, Chatterjee P, Bhatnagar T, Malhotra P, *et al.* Convalescent plasma in the management of moderate COVID-19 in adults in India: open label phase II multicentre randomised controlled trial (PLACID Trial). *BMJ.* 2020;371: m3939.
2. Beigel JH, Tomashek KM, Dodd LE, Mehta AK, Zingman BS, Kalil AC, *et al.* Remdesivir for the Treatment of Covid-19 - Final Report. *N Engl J Med.* 2020;383(19):1813–26.
3. Bernal JL, Andrews N, Gower C, Gallagher E, Simmons R, Thelwall S, et al. Effectiveness of COVID-19 vaccines against the B.1.617.2 variant. *bioRxiv* [Preprint]. 2021. [cited 11 Jul 2021]
4. Budhiraja S, Indrayan A, Aggarwal M, Jha V, Jain D, Tarai B, *et al.* Differentials in the characteristics of COVID-19 cases in Wave-1 and Wave-2 admitted to a network of hospitals in North India. *bioRxiv* [Preprint]. 2021 [cited 11 Jul 2021]
5. Caly L, Druce JD, Catton MG, Jans DA, Wagstaff KM. The FDA-approved drug ivermectin inhibits the replication of SARS-CoV-2 *in vitro. Antiviral Res.* 2020;178:104787.
6. Ella R, Reddy S, Blackwelder W, Potdar V, Yadav P, Sarangi V, et al. Efficacy, safety, and lot to lot immunogenicity of an inactivated SARS-CoV-2 vaccine (BBV152): a, double-blind, randomised, controlled phase 3 trial. *bioRxiv* [Preprint]. 2021. [cited 11 Jul 2021]
7. Gao J, Tian Z, Yang X. Breakthrough: chloroquine phosphate has shown apparent efficacy in treatment of COVID-19 associated pneumonia in clinical studies. *Biosci Trends.* 2020;14(1):72–3.
8. Gautret P, Lagier JC, Parola P, Hoang VT, Meddeb L, Sevestre J, *et al.* Clinical and microbiological effect of a combination of hydroxychloroquine and azithromycin in 80 COVID-19 patients with at least a six-day follow up: a pilot observational study. *Travel Med Infect Dis.* 2020;34:101663.
9. Gordon AC, Mouncey PR, Al-Beidh F, Rowan KM, Nichol AD, Arabi YM, *et al.* Interleukin-6 Receptor Antagonists in Critically Ill Patients with Covid-19. *N Engl J Med.* 2021;384(16): 1491–1502.
10. Horby P, Lim WS, Emberson JR, Mafham M, Bell JL, Linsell L, *et al.* Dexamethasone in Hospitalized Patients with Covid-19. *N Engl J Med.* 2021;384(8):693–704.
11. Iftimie S, López-Azcona AF, Vallverdú I, Hernández-Flix S, de Febrer G, Parra S, *et al.* First and second waves of coronavirus disease-19: A comparative study in hospitalized patients in Reus, Spain. *PLoS One.* 2021;16(3):e0248029.

12. Kalil AC, Patterson TF, Mehta AK, Tomashek KM, Wolfe CR, Ghazaryan V, *et al.* Baricitinib plus Remdesivir for Hospitalized Adults with Covid-19. *N Engl J Med.* 2021;384(9):795–807.

13. Kumar G, Mukherjee A, Sharma RK, Menon GR, Sahu D, Wig N, *et al.* Clinical profile of hospitalized COVID-19 patients in first and second wave of the pandemic: Insights from an Indian registry based observational study. *Indian J Med Res* [Preprint]. 2021 [cited 11 Jul 2021]

14. Pan H, Peto R, Henao-Restrepo AM, Preziosi MP, Sathiyamoorthy V, Abdool Karim Q, *et al.* Repurposed Antiviral Drugs for Covid-19 - Interim WHO Solidarity Trial Results. *N Engl J Med.* 2021;384(6):497–511.

15. Patel A, Agarwal R, Rudramurthy SM, Shevkani M, Xess I, Sharma R, *et al.* Multicenter Epidemiologic Study of Coronavirus Disease-Associated Mucormycosis, India. *Emerg Infect Dis.* 2021;27(9).

16. Schrezenmeier E, Dörner T. Mechanisms of action of hydroxychloroquine and chloroquine: implications for rheumatology. *Nat Rev Rheumatol.* 2020;16(3):155–66.

17. Voysey M, Clemens SAC, Madhi SA, Weckx LY, Folegatti PM, Aley PK, *et al.* Safety and efficacy of the ChAdOx1 nCoV-19 vaccine (AZD1222) against SARS-CoV-2: an interim analysis of four randomised controlled trials in Brazil, South Africa, and the UK. *Lancet.* 2021;397(10269): 99–111.

18. Wei Q, Lin H, Wei RG, Chen N, He F, Zou DH, et al. Tocilizumab treatment for COVID-19 patients: a systematic review and meta-analysis. *Infect Dis Poverty.* 2021;10(1):71.

19. Weinreich DM, Sivapalasingam S, Norton T, Ali S, Gao H, Bhore R, *et al.* REGN-COV2, a Neutralizing Antibody Cocktail, in Outpatients with Covid-19. *N Engl J Med.* 2021;384(3): 238–51.

Psychological Aspects of COVID-19 Pandemic

Kartik Singhai

INTRODUCTION

Extensive research and experience have concurred that psychological ill-effects are widely encountered in pandemic situations such as the current COVID-19 outbreak. The situation is overwhelming for most, more for certain populations than the other. Common mental disorders such as depressive and anxiety disorders as well as post-traumatic stress disorder show an increase in incidence. Apart from diagnosable disorders, the spectrum of emotional distress looms large during such times. Pandemic situations when it comes to mental health response has certain exclusive features such as limited time for planning and prognostication, increased mental health burden on health workers, quarantine, neuropsychiatric sequelae among survivors, dicey status of healthcare facilities.

As with an infectious disease which brings its own pathogens, vectors and mode of transmissions the psychological aspects of the outbreak have their seeds of mis-information, uncertainty and doubt. The stigma and isolation of mental illness coupled with that of the infectious disease become highly burdensome.

Here we shall discuss a few important psychological aspects of the COVID-19 situation.

QUARANTINE AND ITS PSYCHOLOGICAL IMPACT

Quarantine is the separation and restriction of movement of people who have potentially been exposed to a contagious disease with the aim of reducing the risk of them infecting others. This definition is different from an interchangeable used term isolation, which is the separation of people who have been diagnosed with a contagious disease from people who are not sick.

Quarantine is often a displeasing experience. Triggering situations such separation from loved ones, the loss of freedom, uncertainty over disease status, and boredom bear the potential to give rise to varying magnitudes of emotional distress. Studies have shown heightened negative responses such as fear, nervousness, sadness and anger among those quarantined due to being in close contact of positive cases.

Stressors during the quarantine period include duration of quarantine, fear of infection, inadequate supplies, frustration and boredom, inadequate information. Post quarantine, the financial loss can be a problem, with people unable to work and having to interrupt their professional activities with no advanced planning; the effects appear to be long-lasting. Also, stigma is likely to be highly reported among quarantined people with them at risk of facing rejection from local neighborhoods.

COVID-19, HEALTHCARE WORKERS (HCW) AND MENTAL HEALTH

Thousands of healthcare workers across the world form an indispensable core of the frontline against the COVID-19 pandemic. They form one of the most vulnerable populations with regards to mental health issues. The National Institute of Mental Health and Neurosciences, Bengaluru formed a comprehensive report on the same. Common sources of anxiety include fear of exposure to self and transmitting to family, lack of personal protection equipment, lack of information and communication, fear of family welfare if requiring quarantine/isolation. Common manifestations include burn out, distress related to COVID-19, substance use disorder and sleep disturbances.

The sudden reversal of role from HCW to a patient might lead to frustration, helplessness, adjustment issues, stigma, fear of discrimination in the medical staff. Looking at the more optimistic aspects, reviews suggest that social support given to medical staff caused a reduction in anxiety and stress levels and increased self-efficacy of HCW.

Coping measures used by medical staff generally include strict protective measures, knowledge of virus prevention and transmission, social isolation measures, positive self-attitude and social support.

STRATEGIES FOR MENTAL WELL-BEING

The World Health Organization released a report on mental health and psychosocial considerations during the COVID-19 outbreak. Some of the measures suggested in brief included minimizing watching, reading or listening to news about COVID-19 that causes one to feel anxious or distressed; using helpful coping strategies (for HCW) such as ensuring sufficient rest and respite during work or between shifts, eating sufficient and healthy food, engage in physical activity, and staying in contact with family and friends; ensuring good quality communication and accurate information updates, use of psychological first aid.

Special measures for carers of children included helping children find positive ways to express feelings such as fear and sadness, keeping children close to their parents and family and to maintain familiar routines in daily life as much as possible.

MITIGATING THE PSYCHOLOGICAL EFFECTS OF SOCIAL ISOLATION DURING THE COVID-19 PANDEMIC

It is essential to identify and manage adults impacted by the psychological effects of social isolation during the COVID-19 pandemic, and to mitigate the adverse effects of physical distancing. An appropriate approach to the same may include adequate screening for depression, anxiety and loneliness.

People at risk of psychological harm from social isolation during the COVID-19 pandemic include people with pre-existing physical and mental health conditions, older people living alone or in institutions such, disabled individuals, people with substance use disorders, individuals with caretaking responsibilities, people facing unemployment.

The WHO advice for people in isolation includes staying connected and maintaining social networks, paying attention to own needs and feelings, regular mental and physical exercises.

Evidence based strategies for dealing with mental health issues includes the use of online, self-guided cognitive behavioral therapy (CBT), the efficacy of which is well established and at least as effective as face-to-face CBT for many mental health conditions, including anxiety and depression. Two additional evidence-based strategies could reduce psychological harm during the pandemic: remote telephone or video consultations and social prescribing. Telephone consulting is a familiar tool that has been widely used in primary care for decades but is limited by the lack of non-verbal cues. Video consultations provide therapeutic presence and additional visual information and may be particularly useful for anxious patients. Social prescribing is the use of non-medical interventions such as the arts, physical activity, or other community engagement to address broader determinants of health and improve well-being by drawing on existing assets and resources in communities.

Logistics and Economics of Oxygen Usage during COVID Pandemic

Munisha Agarwal, Gunjan Manchanda, Vandana Saith, Farah Husain

The second COVID wave brought with it a deluge of patients which flooded nearly all the hospitals countrywide. The health infrastructure literally collapsed leaving behind a trail of misery and helplessness at all fronts. Much of this was attributed to inadequate medical oxygen infrastructure. We at Lok Nayak Hospital also went through that crisis period in April and May this year, faced several problems but solved them to a large extent and in the process learnt a lot many things which will help us to be better prepared for the anticipated third COVID wave. This chapter aims to share with its readers all the bad that we faced and the good that we learnt.

Learning objectives

- Describe various sources of oxygen available in a hospital including advantages and disadvantages of each.
- Understand how to calculate the daily oxygen demand of a hospital with measures to balance the supply chain accordingly.
- Recognize the challenges faced and the lessons learnt during COVID pandemic at Lok Nayak Hospital.

SOURCES OF OXYGEN IN A HOSPITAL

Factors Determining the Source of Oxygen in a Hospital

A hospital can arrange for a particular type of source of oxygen depending on the following:
1. The calculated consumption pattern of the hospital depending on the bed strength to be equipped with oxygen.
2. The available infrastructure in the premises (central pipeline) and trained technical staff.
3. The dedicated space available in an open area away from inflammable devices such as diesel generators.
4. A reliable supply chain with a vendor.
5. An uninterrupted electric power supply with stabilizer.
6. Cost—capital investment involved and running cost of the oxygen source.
7. Total storage capacity of the source (in metric tons).
8. The availability of a maintenance team of service engineers.

Categories of Sources of Oxygen

- **Primary source:** The primary source of supply shall be permanently connected and shall be the main source of oxygen supply system. As a minimum, the primary supply should have usable quantity of product to meet expected usage between scheduled product deliveries. Primary supply is usually done by liquid medical oxygen (LMO) tank or jumbo gas cylinders using manifold system.
- **Secondary source:** The secondary source of supply shall be permanently connected, automatically supply the pipeline and capable of providing the total oxygen flow requirement in the event of a primary failure. As a minimum, the secondary supply should have usable quantity of product to meet expected usage between a request for product delivery and the delivery of the product.
- **Reserve or backup** supply at source or bedside: The reserve supply is the final source of supply to specific sections of the pipeline, capable of meeting the required demand in the event of failure of the primary and secondary supplies, or failure of the upstream distribution pipe work. As a minimum, the reserve supply should have usable quantity of product to meet critical patient care between a request for product delivery and the delivery of the product. Under most conditions, compressed gas cylinders are the most appropriate method of providing a reserve source of supply.

Types of Oxygen Sources in a Hospital

Every source has certain advantages and disadvantages, and if we consider all the above-mentioned points while installing a source, we would be able to manage high oxygen demand scenarios with coordinated teamwork between doctors, technicians, suppliers and service engineers.

The different types of sources available for any hospital comprise of:
1. Liquid oxygen tank
2. PSA plant (oxygen generator)
3. Cylinders (manifold in gas plant room and bedside)
4. Oxygen concentrators (bedside).

TABLE 19.1: Description of various sources of oxygen in a hospital

Type of source	Working principle	Applications and uses	Advantages	Disadvantages
Liquid oxygen (LOX) plant **Fig. 19.1:** LOX tank with 2 vaporizers (*Source:* Lok Nayak Hospital, New Delhi)	LOX is generated outside hospital at large plants called air separation units	Applications and uses for all types of oxygen supplies in the hospital (ICU, OT, wards including high flow oxygen)	Advantages no electrical supply is needed	Requires very reliable supply and transport chain
	Fractional distillation of air to derive liquefied oxygen by reducing boiling point of oxygen gas to less than 182°C	It is distributed by the pipeline system, and provided bedside in the various wards by wall outlet points	Oxygen can be provided even at high flows	Exhaustible supply that needs adequate infrastructure and pipeline system

(Contd.)

TABLE 19.1: Description of various sources of oxygen in a hospital (Contd.)

Type of source	Working principle	Applications and uses	Advantages	Disadvantages
Fig. 19.2: Outlets from the LOX tank going to the vaporizer with ice crystals and the open outlet for refilling of tank (*Source:* Lok Nayak Hospital, New Delhi)	Stored in LOX storage tank that is vertically installed, after obtaining a PESO license at a barricaded area in the hospital. Medical oxygen is produced as LOX moves into air heated vaporizers an is distributed through pipelines in the hospital	Highest purity of oxygen is given 99%	Requires a small space for installation	Needs trained technical staff for up keep. Risk of gas leakage through pipeline. Requires backup supply of cylinders
PSA (pressure swing adsorption) plant (Oxygen generator) Fig. 19.3: Air receiving tank (*Source:* PSA plant at Lok Nayak Hospital, New Delhi) Fig. 19.4: Moisture and the dust filters attached to the air dryer (*Source:* PSA plant at Lok Nayak Hospital, New Delhi)	An onsite oxygen generating plant up to 5000 L/min. Four steps in process of oxygen generation by the PSA plant 1. Compressed air is taken into the air receiving tank, cooled and dried and after filtration of dust and moisture, it is passed onto the generator with zeolite membranes for adsorption of nitrogen 2. Production of oxygen after concentrating it from the atmospheric air and passing it inside the oxygen product tank, and passed into the pipeline after the final activated carbon filter 3. Switch and blow out: As first membrane gets exhausted with nitrogen, compressed air inlet is switched to the second generator side as blow out of other gases from the first membrane occurs through an exhaust 4. Purging of the first membrane to keep it ready for the next switch. This is an automatic process	For all oxygen supplies in the hospital. It is distributed by the pipeline system, and provided in the various wards by wall outlet points. Purity of oxygen is given 90–95%. Can generate between 100 5000 L/min of oxygen. Can be used to fill oxygen cylinders using a booster compressor within the hospital premises	For all oxygen supplies in the hospital through a pipeline system. Continuous supply of oxygen is available in the hospital. A PSA plant is an on-site production as well as a storage unit. It does not depend on any external supply chain	Needs a stable and uninterrupted electrical power supply. Needs an initially high capital investment. Requires significant area in the hospital and a specifically designed room. Needs highly trained staff for maintenance. Risk of gas leakage through the pipeline. Needs backup cylinder supply

(Contd.)

TABLE 19.1: Description of various sources of oxygen in a hospital (Contd.)

Type of source	Working principle	Applications and uses	Advantages	Disadvantages

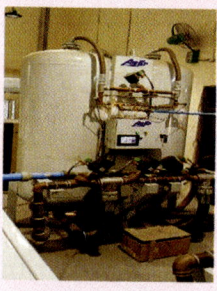

Fig. 19.5: Generators with zeolite membrane and outlets going to the oxygen product tank (*Source:* PSA plant at Lok Nayak Hospital, New Delhi)

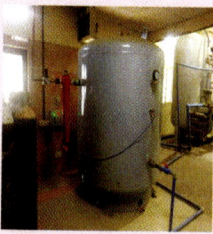

Fig. 19.6: Oxygen product Tank with the activated carbon filter (red) attached to its outlet from where oxygen is then moved into the pipeline system. (*Source:* PSA plant at Lok Nayak Hospital, New Delhi)

Cylinders

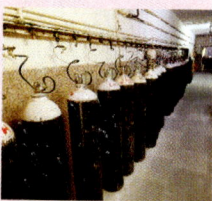

Fig. 19.7: Oxygen cylinder banks (left and right) at the gas manifold made up of 6–20 D type cylinders to supply oxygen through pipeline as a back up (*Source:* Gas Plant at Lok Nayak Hospital, New Delhi)

A refillable cylindrical storage vessel used to store and transport oxygen in compressed gas form

They are refilled at off-site gas generating plant and thus require transportation to and from the plant

D type–used in manifolds at the gas plant

For all oxygen supplies in wards

At the manifold used as back up for other primary sources

Regular checks of oxygen levels in cylinder by pressure gauge and cleaning of cylinder exterior and disinfection as they were returned from COVID wards

Limited maintenance required by trained technicians

No electrical power source needed

Provides emergency back-up facility at hospitals to other primary sources

Requires a very reliable transport/supply chain

Exhaustible supply

Highly reliant upon supplier

Risk of gas leakage and damage of safety valves during transport

(Contd.)

TABLE 19.1: Description of various sources of oxygen in a hospital (Contd.)

Type of source	Working principle	Applications and uses	Advantages	Disadvantages
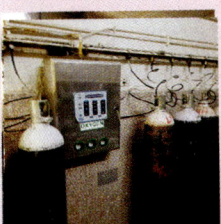 **Fig. 19.8:** Oxygen control panel that allows the automatic switch between the left and the right banks (*Source:* **Gas** Plant at Lok Nayak Hospital, New Delhi)	Contains 7000 L of compressed medical oxygen B type–used bedside and in transport Contains 1500 L of compressed medical oxygen A type–used as backup for the anesthesia workstations in operation theaters Contains 690 L of oxygen	The automatic oxygen control panel at the manifold enables the switch over between right and left bank Emergency manifolds can be created with smaller number of D type cylinders in the wards Bedside use of B type cylinders as a backup supply		
Oxygen concentrator 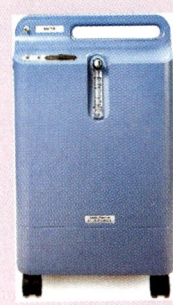 **Fig. 19.9:** Bedside oxygen concentrator (*Source:* Creative commons)	It is like a smaller, compact PSA plant A self-contained, electrically powered medical device designed to concentrate oxygen from ambient air, using PSA technology Oxygen concentration of about 90–95% can be produced This bedside piece of equipment has following parts 1. Compressor to pressurize atmospheric air and draw it into the concentrator 2. A heat exchanger to reduce the temperature of this pressurised air 3. A surge tank to store this air 4. 2 zeolite molecular sieves to adsorb nitrogen 5. A product tank 6. Outlet with a flowmeter 7. Humidifcation chamber 8. Filter Directly provides oxygen to the patient with tubing through a flowmeter @ 1–10 L/minute	Depending on weight of machine 1. Small (5–10 kg) have small compressors: FiO_2 decreases from 90% to 30% as flows increase from 1 to 9 L/minute. It is not suitable for COVID patients (COPD patients can use) 2. Medium (15–19 kg) concentrators–have compressors can easily give an output of 90% oxygen @1–5 L/minute may be used in mild-moderate COVID disease 3. Large (≥20 kg) concentrators, suitable for critical and COVID patients- have large compressors which can give an output of 90% oxygen from 1–10 LPM flow. Ideal for COVID patients and critical care patients and for dual patients to use same machine with accessories	Used to deliver oxygen at the bedside using mask or nasal prongs Continuous oxygen supply (if power available) at low running cost Output flow can be split among 2 patients with a large concentrator Can be used in pediatric and adult population depending on the output	Low pressure output, usually not suitable for CPAP or ventilators Requires uninterrupted power Requires backup cylinder supply Requires moderate amount of maintenance–re-filling of the humidification chamber and filter changes Needs distilled water for humidification

MATHEMATICS OF OXYGEN DEMAND AND SUPPLY

Mathematics of liquid oxygen is complex yet interesting. "We are consuming oxygen in liters, storing it in KL, paying in kg or m^3 and projecting our demand in MT." Thus, we must understand and remember these unit conversions. For calculation of O_2 demand we should know the consumption of O_2 in a hospital in a day. The oxygen capacity of the hospital's source should be such that they are able to meet the peak oxygen demand. The dealing of liquid oxygen in day-to-day life requires knowledge of various unit conversions of oxygen. The common conversions used are summarized in Fig. 19.10.

LMO Vessel

LMO storage capacity of LMO vessels: The capacities of LMO vessels varies from 1 KL to 1500 KL. The density of the liquid oxygen is 1.1417 kg/L or 1141.7 kg/m^3 (1 m^3 = 1000 L).

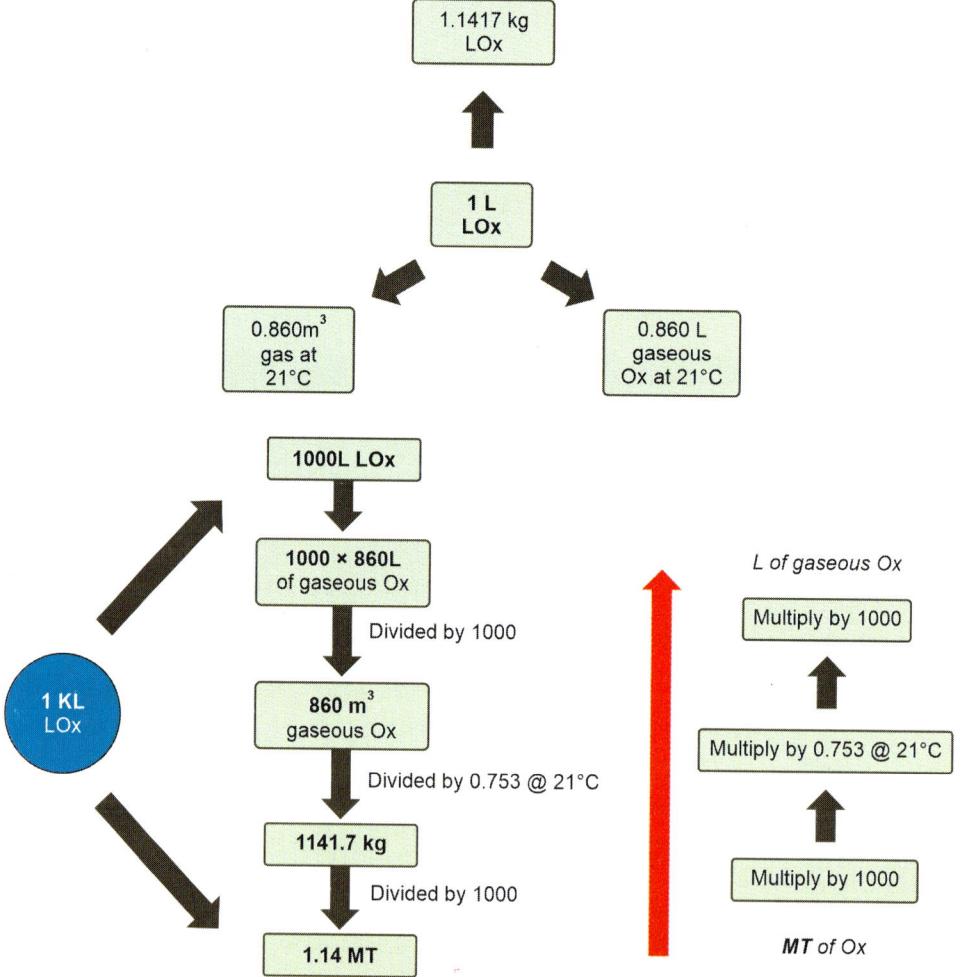

Fig. 19.10: Common conversions used in oxygen gas management

It is to be noted that no LMO vessels are filled till brim. They are not filled to full capacity. The vessels are at the maximum filled up to 90% of their defined capacities. For example, if a hospital say, Lok Nayak Hospital has two LMO vessels with capacity of 16 KL and 10 KL. Let us calculate the usable storage capacities of the liquid medical oxygen in this hospital. For the first LMO vessel of total defined capacity of 16 KL the total usable storage capacity shall be 14.4 KL (90% of 16 KL) and for the second vessel with total defined capacity of 10 KL it shall be 9.0 KL. Hence the total storage capacity of LMO for this hospital is 23.4 KL. Now, this can also be obtained from the LMO vendor who provide the charts where it is mentioned about the total capacity for filling up of vessel.

Calculation the time for LMO vessel to be refilled: It is important to consider and prepare the facility with the appropriate time management for timely replenishment of LMO to ensure uninterrupted supply of oxygen in a healthcare facility. When should these vessels should be refilled? In general, vessel must be refilled when oxygen left in vessel is 25% of capacity. This is also known as 'reserve capacity' of the LMO vessel. The calculations regarding time to refill of a LMO vessel is exemplified in Fig. 19.11.

Scenario #1: *A hospital has daily consumption of 5000 LPM of oxygen. For how many hours this LMO vessel of 16 KL will last?*
- Total vessel capacity = 16 KL
- Maximum usable LMO available
- 16 KL × 90% = 14.4 KL
- Time the usable liquid oxygen shall last can be calculated as follows:
  - As consumption of O_2 in the hospital is 5000 L/minute
  - Total available LMO = 14.4 KL (if the vessel is filled to the maximum usable limits)

Using the formula:

$$\text{Time the usable oxygen shall last} = \frac{\text{Available gaseous oxygen in L} \times \text{gaseous oxygen per liter}}{\text{Oxygen consumption (LPM)}}$$

- (14.4 × 1000 × 860)/5000
- = 2476.8 min = ~41 hours
- Reserve is 3.5 KL (25% of total usable capacity)
- (3500 × 860)/5000 = 602 min = ~10 hours.

Fig. 19.11: The real-life scenario on how to calculate time to refill of a LMO vessel

LMO capacity measurements in real-time: In a typical LMO vessel at least two gauge are mounted to monitor amount of LMO present in the vessel and the pressure of the vessel outlet. The first gauge which monitors content of the vessel shows amount of LMO in the vessel in mm of water column (mmWC) (Fig. 19.12). The second gauge shows vessel pressure in bars or pressure per square inch (psi).

Let us examine a scenario, wherein if the LMO tank has readings as shown in Fig. 19.3, how long will the LMO vessel last? The calculations are summarized in Fig. 19.13.

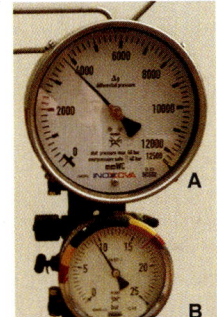

Fig. 19.12: The volume gauge and the pressure gauge mounted on the LMO vessels: (A) Volume gauge; (B) Pressure gauge

If actual reading of an LMO vessel is as shown in Fig. 19.3 above, let us calculate. How many hours this vessel will last?

- Oxygen level on the gauge A is **3800 mm WC** = 7140 L (Liquid oxygen) = 6262 m³ (gaseous O_2) at 27°C (as per conversion chart provided by the supplier).
- As 1 m³ = 1000 L so to convert 6262 m³ to liters we have to multiply it with 1000
  - 6262 m³ × 1000 = 6262000 L of (gaseous O_2) at 27°C
  - Assuming hospital oxygen consumption is 5000 L/minute
  - 6262000L/5000 L/min = ~1252 minutes = ~20 hours.
  - This vessel with consumption of 5000 L/minute shall last 20 hours.

Fig. 19.13: Calculations regarding capacities and pressure in LMO vessel and its relation to the emptying time

Oxygen Cylinders

These are another important source of oxygen in a hospital. The different types of cylinders commonly available in the hospital are described elsewhere. Among these D-type and B-type cylinders are the one which are common to provide acute care services in the hospital. Their capacities and conversions are summarized in Table 19.1. The D-type cylinders are the key storing capacities among all types and is also used in cylinder manifold installed in the hospital.

TABLE 19.1: Capacity and conversion of oxygen cylinder

Cylinder type	Capacity in liters	Capacity in CuM (mm³)	Capacity in kg	Capacity in MT
D Type	7000	7(7000/1000)	9.94(7 × 1.3)	0.00995(9.95/1000)
B Type	1500	1.5(1500/1000)	2.13(1.5 × 1.3)	0.00213(2.13/1000)

At 1 atmosphere, Temperature 21°C

Now let us examine a scenario wherein *if a D-type cylinder is connected to a patient with oxygen requirement of 10 L/minute, how much time is required to get the cylinder empty?* We know, capacity of a D-type cylinder is 7000 L and flow rate for oxygen delivery is 10 L/minute, hence, time required to get the cylinder empty = 7000/10= 700 minutes = 11.6 hours.

It is necessary to emphasize here that B-type cylinders are used for patient transport with oxygen. These cylinders should not be part of calculations towards covid dedicated hospital's oxygen storage capacity. These are the cylinders which are used to carry patients on oxygen in ambulance as well hence the time to empty of the cylinders are important to calculate to determine the cylinders to be carried during patient transport to ensure uninterrupted oxygen supply to the patients. The example of such scenario is described in Fig. 19.14.

- We know, capacity of a B-type cylinder is 1500 L and there the flow rate is 5 L/minute
- Hence, time required to get the cylinder empty = 1500 L/5 LPM = 300 minutes = 5 hours
- Thus, this ambulance should carry patient with at least two B-type cylinders.

Fig. 19.14: If a patient with oxygen requirement of 5 L/minute is connected to a B-type cylinder, and this patient is required to be transported from remote area which will take 6 hours to reach hospital, how many such cylinders an ambulance should carry?

Cylinder Manifold

A typical manifold has two banks (left bank and right banks). One bank is used as a backup of other bank. Thus, if one bank is empty, the supply switch to the other bank and alarm the operator to replace the cylinders of the emptied side. The two banks generally have 6 to 14 oxygen cylinders each. There can be larger banks as per requirements of the hospitals. Typically, the cylinder manifold is the backup supply for LMO supply in a healthcare setting. Higher cylinder capacity of the manifold does not necessarily mean higher oxygen output capacity of a manifold. The oxygen output from the manifold depends upon regulator mounted on the control panel which regulates flow and pressure in the gas pipeline connected to a manifold. The control panels with flow rates of 1100, 1500, 2000 LPM, etc. are available which delivers oxygen at 60 psi. Now let us examine how to ensure number of cylinders required to be used a back up to LMO supply (Fig. 19.15).

- Now, 2 MT LMO is consumed in 24 hours
  = 2 MT = 2000 kg
- As 1L LMO = 1.1417 kg
  2000 kg = 2000/1.1417 = 1751 L LOX
- 1L LOX = 860 L gaseous O_2
  Thus 1751 L LOX × 860 = 1505860 L gaseous O_2 in 24 hours = 1505860/24 × 60 ~ 1045 LPM
- Therefore, oxygen consumption = 1045 L/minute
- Now, if the hospital has 6 × 6-cylinder manifold as a backup for 2 MT supply in 24 hours it shall be supplying 1045 L/minute
- The one oxygen bank of 6 cylinders shall last = 6 × 7000/1045 = 40 minutes [approx.]
  Thus, in 1440 minutes (24 hours) number of cylinders required (1440/40) × 6 = 216 cylinders.

Fig. 19.15: If a hospital has 2MT LMO consumption which is not available due to supply chain or technical issues—how many D-type cylinders are required to run the manifold to get this 2MT oxygen?

Oxygen Generator/Concentrators

There are two types of systems available in the hospital where oxygen can be generated at hospital level. The first is pressure swing adsorption plant (PSA) and the other one is portable oxygen concentrator.

Oxygen generator/concentrator (PSA plants): In this type of systems oxygen generated is measured in liters per minutes (LPM) or m^3/hour. It is available in various capacities and can be installed as per requirement of the hospital. It is to be emphasized here, that PSA runs on electric supply and have oxygen purity of less than 95% hence they are not suitable to be used as primary source of oxygen supplies in critical care units of the hospitals. It is important to relate the capacity of a PSA plant with the total oxygen generated in units it is used at patient level to understand flow rate from the PSA (Fig. 19.16).

- **We know 1 m^3/hour = 1000 L/hour**
- Hence, 90 m^3/hour = 90 × 1000 = 90,000 L/hour = 90,000/60 = 1500 LPM

Fig. 19.16: If capacity of PSA plant is 90 m^3/hour. How much oxygen the plant can deliver in LPM?

Portable oxygen concentrators (POCs): These generate small quantity of oxygen flow, usually 2–5 LPM. The total capacity calculated by multiplying the available number of concentrators with generation capacity, e.g. if we have 100 concentrators of 5 LPM then total capacity shall be = 100×5 LPM = 500 LPM. Total capacity per day (24 hours) can be calculated as follows: 500 LPM = $500 \times 60 \times 24$ = 720000 L/day = 720000/1000 m^3/day = 720 m^3/day

720 m^3/day = 720/0.77 = 935 kg/day

Thus, 935 kg/1000 = 0.935 MT/day

Hence, the total capacity of these 100 POCs with capacity of 5 LPM is 0.935 MT/day.

The total oxygen consumption in a dedicated covid hospital can be calculated using either of the following methods:

a. Based on oxygen devices distribution among critical care units and other non-ICU patient care units.

b. Based on disease severity (severe cases and critical cases).

c. Based location and distribution.

With the information as discussed above about the various oxygen sources and conversions, let us examine a scenario of a dedicated covid hospital (Fig. 19.17).

Hence, no matter which method among the three methods described in Fig. 19.8 is used, usage of oxygen devices (~2.851 MT), patients with disease severity (~2.805 MT) bed location and distribution (~2.524 MT). The oxygen requirement is similar. It is important to note that monitoring high consumption areas on daily basis is recommended to improve oxygen consumption in the hospital.

It is further recommended that the projected oxygen demand should be of minimum 72 hours, ideally 5–7 days. In the special situations like pandemic and disaster, if supply constrains are present a minimum of 24 hours demand should be available. Major factor when arranging the oxygen supplies is the lead time. The lead time in case of LMO supply is the time taken between raising the demand to the supplier to initiation of vessel filling. In case of cylinder supplies is time taken between raising the demand to the supplier to fixation of cylinders to the manifold. It varies from institution-to-institution and also varies with supplier (few institutions may have more than one vendor).

Finally, the projected demand should be sum total of buffer capacity of LMO vessel (25% of total storage capacity of vessel), oxygen consumption during lead time and actual oxygen consumption. If the buffer capacity is available, the total demand shall be sum total of lead time and actual oxygen consumption.

Conclusions

Oxygen conversion formulae are critical for day-to-day management of oxygen supply and demand in a hospital setting. The oxygen consumption and requirement are similar no matter which of the three methods discussed are used. Close monitoring of high oxygen consumption areas is required when calculating oxygen requirement on daily basis. Alternate sources of oxygen must be present with adequate capacity and tested on periodic basis.

The oxygen consumption depends on the number of different devices used in a hospital. The flow rates are being used as recommended by WHO.

Let us estimate the total estimated oxygen consumption in this hospital.

Device	Bed distribution (100 bedded hosp)	Anticipated consumption (LPM)	Total O_2 consumption (L/day)
Ventilator	05	10	10 × 05 × 1440 = 72000
HFNO	10	60	60 × 10 × 1440 = 864000
NIV/BIPAP	10	15	15 × 10 × 1440 = 216000
NRBM/venturi mask	30	15	15 × 30 × 1440 = 648000
Nasal prongs	35	05	5 × 35 × 1440 = 252000
Face mask	10	10	10 × 10 × 1440 = 144000
Total oxygen consumption			**21,96,000 L/day**

It is to be noted that this is equipment-based calculations. The number of devices which use higher oxygen should be kept closely monitored for variation in oxygen consumption. Also, *1 day = 24 hours = 24 x 60 minutes = 1440 minutes* has been used in the calculations above.

- Thus, the total consumption = 2196000 **L/day**
  = 2196 m³ (2196000/**1000**) = 2851 **kg** (2196/**0.77**)
  = 2.851 **MT** (2851/**1000**) = **2.49 KL** (2.851/**1.1417**) *(as 1 KL = 1.14 MT)*
  Now, this should be 90% of total storage capacity of LMO vessel
- Thus, vessel capacity of at least 3–4 KL is required for this hospital (assuming this shall be filled on daily basis)
- Thus, if the vessel needs to be filled once in three days (72 hours), the vessel of **capacity 9–12 KL is required**

Now, let us calculate oxygen requirement based on disease severity in this hospital.

Disease severity	Average O_2 flow rate (LPM)		Anticipated O_2 consumption (L/day)
	Per patient	Total	
Severe (75)	**10 LPM**	75 × 10 = 750	750 × 60 × 24 = 10,80,000
Critical (25)	**30 LPM**	25 × 30 = 750	750 × 60 × 24 = 10,80,000
Total oxygen consumption			**21,60,000**

(Based on oxygen sources and distribution for COVID 19 treatment centers. Interim Guidance. World Health Organization. April 4 2020)

- Thus, the total O_2 consumption = 21,60,000 L/day
  = 2160 m³ (2160000/1000) = 2805 **kg** (2160/0.77)
  = 2.805 **MT** (2805/1000) = 2.456 **KL** (2.805/1.1417)

Another method to calculate the oxygen consumption in a 100 bedded dedicated hospital is calculating the oxygen requirement based on bed location and distribution in the hospital. (This is the method recommended by Ministry of Health and Family Welfare, Govt of India)

Bed types	Average O_2 flow rate (LPM)		Anticipated O_2 consumption (L/day)
	Per patient	Total	
Non-ICU (75)	**10 LPM**	75 × 10 = 750	750 × 60 × 24 = 10,80,000
ICU (25)	**24 LPM**	25 × 24 = 600	600 × 60 × 24 = 8,64,000
Total oxygen consumption			**19,44,000**

- Thus, the total consumption = 19,44,000 L/day
  = 1944 m³ (1944000/1000) = 2524 **kg** (1944/0.77)
  = 2.524 **MT** (2524/1000) = 2.21 **KL** (2.524/1.1417)

Fig. 19.17: In a 100 bedded COVID hospital with various oxygen devices distribution among COVID patients is given. Calculate the total oxygen consumption and LMO vessel capacity required for this hospital.

CHALLENGES FACED AT LOK NAYAK HOSPITAL AND LESSONS LEARNT

COVID-19 pandemic revealed a major weakness in the existing healthcare infrastructure-that of medical oxygen production and delivery. Demand far exceeded the supply making oxygen a precious commodity. We at LNH faced many problems during this pandemic and resolved them to a large extent.

Increase in Number of Oxygen Supported Beds

Lok Nayak Hospital which was declared a COVID dedicated hospital with 2000 beds had central oxygen supply to 500 beds only when the pandemic started. Concerted and coordinated efforts of various departments like PWD, administration, and Anesthesia department were required to quickly establish a central piped oxygen supply to all 2000 beds.

Pipeline Gauge and Pressure Issues

Since many COVID-19 patients required high flow of oxygen (60–70 L/minute), we had to install 28 mm copper pipeline (earlier laid pipeline was of 22 mm bore) in the wards while at the source pipeline as wide as 54 mm and 42 mm diameter was required to achieve the high flow of oxygen at the required pressure.

Placement of isolation valves at strategic points on the pipeline had to be planned. This ensured that supply of oxygen to other parts of the building continued uninterrupted while repair work was on. Now, that the pipelines were laid to meet the growing demand, some modifications were also made in the main pipeline exiting from the primary source, i.e. LMO vessel. High pressure regulators (100 kg/cm^2 supplying 1667 L/minute) were replaced with regulator of 250 kg/cm^2 to supply at 4000 L/minute at the LMO tanks to meet the high flow demand of oxygen.

LMO Vessel and Cylinders

Additional bigger vaporizer providing 1200 m^3/hour of oxygen in addition to old vaporizer providing 400 m^3/hour of oxygen was installed so that they could convert higher quantity of liquid oxygen into oxygen gas to meet the demand for higher flow rates of oxygen. While this work was to be done, oxygen supply from LMO tank was shut and we had to use the standby sources like manifolds and a bypass system between the two LMO vessels of the hospital to maintain supply of oxygen to the wards and ICUs during the repair period.

The second wave of the pandemic was different from the first wave in many respects—main difference being the huge number of patients admitted to the hospital in just a short span of time leading to massive surge in oxygen demand. This in turn led to gross imbalance in demand supply ratio of oxygen.

There was a severe shortage of supply of liquid medical oxygen and oxygen cylinders. On one hand, we were witness to rapidly depleting oxygen levels in LMO tank while on the other we had to struggle with vendors to send their LMO supply on time. LMO vessels which required refilling only once a week during pre-COVID times, now required to be filled twice daily! Refilling of cylinders was required at much faster rate. There were long queues at the filling stations which led to delay in fresh supply of oxygen cylinders reaching the hospital. With the crucial LMO being in short supply, we had to take urgent measures to get our empty cylinders refilled at the earliest like hiring our own vehicles and sending technicians along with the vehicles to ensure refilling at the earliest. Such was the shortage of oxygen that the vehicles and staff had to wait in queue at the filling stations for 48–72 hours. Taking cognisance of the situation, the Delhi Government designated multiple cylinder filling vendors for each hospital which eased out the problem.

The government also started sending us oxygen supplies through SOS oxygen tankers which would refill LMO in minimal quantity to help us tide over the period till our designated vendor sent the LMO supply. Another small big problem that we encountered was incompatibility of adapter connection of cryogenic tankers and LMO vessel. We realized the need for universal adapters/connecters to resolve this issue. To overcome the growing oxygen crisis, a PSA plant of 2000 l/minute capacity was installed to have in-house oxygen generator. 3 more PSA plants are also being installed currently at LNH to ramp up the in-house oxygen generating capacity.

Human Resource

There was scarcity of trained manpower at all levels, i.e. doctors, nurses, technicians, housekeeping staff. To add to our problems, COVID infection was taking toll of our already dwindling staff. Many who were even fully vaccinated were falling prey to this deadly disease. Urgent need for recruitment of staff at all levels was realized and steps to that end were initiated. In house training classes on oxygen therapy and its devices was done. Dedicated teaching training videos were circulated amongst the staff on WhatsApp groups.

Rationalizing the Oxygen Usage

Unanticipated stupendous increase in oxygen consumption leading to gross imbalance between its demand and supply made it imperative to rationalize its usage at all levels.

At Patient Level

1. Target oxygen saturation of the patient to be maintained between 94 and 95%. Do not aim to achieve SpO_2 of 100%.
2. Timely de-escalating oxygen flow rates according to patient's clinical condition.
3. Change of interface or oxygen therapy device itself instead of arbitrarily increasing oxygen flow rates.
4. Ensuring proper fitting masks/interface.
5. Switching off oxygen therapy device when not in use (no use period), e.g. patient goes to washroom, is discharged.
6. Judicious use of high flow oxygen devices (HFNO) in ICU settings and under supervision of pulmonologist/physician.
7. Use of oxygen conserving strategies, e.g. oxymizer nasal cannula, change to proper interface or device.

At Administrative Level

There was an urgent need for "monitoring and analyzing daily oxygen requirement" of the hospital to further rationalize oxygen usage. To this end following steps were suggested:

1. Formulation of 'oxygen monitoring teams' comprising of nurse, technician who will monitor and timely detect any leaky oxygen port, no-use period of oxygen therapy.
2. "Oxygen monitoring committee" comprising of members from hospital administration, anesthesia and medicine departments, nursing superintendent. This committee will be required to properly monitor, analyze and audit daily oxygen requirement of the hospital including demand-supply logistics.
3. Real time digital dashboards to track the oxygen supply through cryogenic tankers and cylinders at a central level.

Rationalizing the usage of oxygen by intense monitoring and auditing both at patient level as well as the supply end will help us to plan and organize our oxygen resources judiciously. We need to estimate our peak projected requirement of oxygen correctly and plan oxygen sources accordingly including adequate buffer stock. Crisis can occur at anytime, what is needed is to be prepared at all times and this requires concerted team effort of clinicians, nurses, technicians, administration and the government.

BIBLIOGRAPHY

1. Amrita.edu. Before you buy oxygen concentrator. May 2021.
2. Blakeman TC, Branson RD. Oxygen Supplies in Disaster Management. Respir Care 2013;58(1):173–82.
3. Graham HR, Bagayana SM, Bakare AA, et al. Improving hospital oxygen systems for COVID-19 in low-resource settings: lessons from the field. Glob Health Sci Pract. 2020;8(4).
4. Oxygen allocation order (PA/SS-II/H and FW/COVID-19/Part IV/ 850 dated 07/05/2021. Government of NCT of Delhi. https://delhi.gov.in/7_05_2021.pdf.
5. Oxygen sources and distribution for COVID-19 treatment centres. Interim guidance. 4 April 2020. WHO/2019-nCoV/Oxygen_sources/2020.1.
6. Uttar Pradesh State Oxygen Operational Guidelines and Guidebook.
7. WHO-UNICEF Technical Specifications and Guidance for Oxygen Therapy Devices. 2019. Available at:https://www.who.int/medical_devices/publications/tech_specs_oxygen_therapy_devices/en/

Hematological Manifestations in COVID-19

Sunita Aggarwal, Sheeba Khan, Sandeep Garg, Kanika Negi

Coronavirus disease (COVID-19) is a multi-systemic infectious disease caused by a newly discovered coronavirus SARS-CoV-2 with an incubation period of 1–14 days. It is currently a pandemic, with more than 185 million cases and roughly 4 million deaths globally as of 9 July 2021, with the United States and India leading the way. The Indian capital Delhi has witnessed 1.4 million cases and 25 thousand deaths. The novel coronavirus, known as severe acute respiratory syndrome coronavirus 2 (SARS-CoV-2), belongs to the beta group of the Coronaviridae family and it is the third well known zoonotic disease of coronaviruses after severe acute respiratory syndrome (SARS-CoV) and middle east respiratory syndrome (MERS-CoV). The SARS-CoV-2 virus that causes COVID-19 is mainly transmitted through droplets generated when an infected person coughs, sneezes, or exhales. Fever, dry cough, and tiredness are common symptoms of COVID-19. However, a subset of patients develops a more severe form of the disease, characterized by acute respiratory distress syndrome (ARDS), neurological, cardiac, and renal, hematopoietic, and immune complications.[1]

HEMATOLOGICAL PROFILE IN COVID-19

During the course of the disease, longitudinal evaluation of hematological parameters such as lymphocyte count dynamics and inflammatory indices, including LDH, CRP, and IL-6 may help to spot cases with dismal prognosis and early intervention to improve outcomes (Table 20.1).

TABLE 20.1: Hematological manifestations of COVID-19	
Lymphopenia (83.2%)	Elevated CRP (60.7%)
Neutrophilia (34.5%)	Procalcitonin (5.5%)
Mild thrombocytopenia (36.2%)	**COVID-19-associated coagulopathy (76%)**
Monocytopenia	Elevated D-Dimers
Elevated LDH	Prolonged PT
Reactive and plasmacytoid lymphocytes on blood film	Prolonged APTT
	Elevated fibrinogen
Elevated ferritin (78.5%)	
Elevated ESR (93.8%)	

MECHANISMS OF SARS-COV-2 INVASION TO HOST CELLS

SARS-CoV-2, similar to SARS-CoV-1, enters the host cells through angiotensin-converting enzyme 2 (ACE2) receptors that are expressed in the alveolar epithelial cells type 2 and 1, myocytes, vascular endothelial cells, hematopoietic stem cells, and progenitors. After attaching to the ACE2 receptors, the spike proteins of SARS-CoV-2 are broken down through acid-dependent proteolysis by cathepsin, transmembrane protease-serine 2 (TMPRSS2) and consequently, the SARS-CoV-2 merges with the cell membrane.[2] Recent studies suggested that SARS-CoV-2 may also attack host cells via the CD147-spike protein (SP) pathway. SP aids the virus invasion by connecting to CD147. CD147 is a plasma membrane protein from the immunoglobulin family and is found in hematopoietic cells, mesenchymal stem cells, leukocytes, epithelial and endothelial cells, and has a variety of physiological and pathological functions.

Studies showed that as CD147 is expressed on the red blood cells (as an adhesion molecule), its role is of vital importance in the circulation of mature red blood cells from the spleen to the bloodstream.[3]

EFFECTS ON RED BLOOD CELLS AND HEMOGLOBIN

Reduced hemoglobin levels have been noted in some severe COVID-19 patients. No significant effects on red blood cell (RBC) counts have been found, but structural changes have been noted with the resultant increase in **red cell distribution width (RDW)**. Red blood cells of COVID-19 patients had increased oxidation of structural proteins and altered lipid metabolism.[4]

PERIPHERAL BLOOD FILM

Examination of the peripheral blood smear reported an increased frequency of reactive and plasmacytoid lymphocytes, significant left-shifted granulopoiesis with hyper granular, occasionally vacuolated neutrophils, and leucoerythroblastic features. The presence of schistocytes or red cell fragments has not been reported.[5]

EFFECTS ON WHITE BLOOD CELLS

Lymphocytes

- Due to the high prevalence of lymphopenia in patients with COVID-19 and its strong association with the severity of the disease, lymphocytes count can be used as a predictive biomarker for the severity of the disease.
- Lymphopenia in these patients leads to a reduction of the total number of lymphocytes, TCD4+, TCD8+, B cells, and natural killer cells (NK cells), which the reduction of CD8+ T cells more significant. Zhao *et al* in a meta-analysis study demonstrated that the risk of severe COVID-19 increased by about threefold in patients with lymphopenia.[6]
- Since lymphocytes express ACE2 and CD147 on their membrane, it is hypothesized that SARS-CoV-2 may directly invade lymphocytes, leading to lysis of lymphocytes and lymphopenia.
- There is a negative relationship between serum levels of interleukin 6 (IL-6), interleukin 10 (IL-10), and tumor necrosis factor-alpha (TNFα) with the number of lymphocytes.

- **The neutrophil-to-lymphocyte ratio (NLR ratio)** was higher in severe COVID-19 patients is calculated by dividing the absolute number of neutrophils by the absolute number of lymphocytes and is of great importance in expressing the general inflammatory condition of the patient.[8]

Neutrophil-to-lymphocyte ratio	NLR
Mild COVID-19	<3.2
Moderate COVID-19	>3.2
Severe COVID-19	>5.5

Currently, corticosteroids are used to reduce COVID-19 related inflammation. Dexamethasone 0.1–0.2 mg/kg or methylprednisolone 0.5–1 mg/kg for 5 days in moderate cases and dexamethasone 0.2 mg/kg–0.4 mg/kg or methylprednisolone 1.0–2.0 mg/kg for 10 days in severe cases.[9]

Neutrophil

- Neutrophilic leukocytosis was linked with a high-risk of the acute respiratory syndrome, risk of death, and elevated troponin levels. In addition, neutrophil infiltration into the pulmonary capillaries, extravasation of neutrophils into the alveolar space, and neutrophilic mucositis were found in the autopsy report of patients with COVID-19.[7]

PLATELETS

- Thrombocytopenia is reported in 5%–40% of patients, and platelet count <200 × 109/L at admission was associated with three times higher mortality although the degree of thrombocytopenia seen is generally mild. Platelet counts were found to decrease from around day 4 of symptoms.[10]
- Mechanisms of development of thrombocytopenia are the direct and indirect effect of SARS-CoV-2 on the hematopoietic cells and endothelial cells, which can be associated with impaired megakaryocyte maturation, increased platelet aggregation, platelet activation, and consequently, platelet consumption in the microcirculation of damaged lung tissue.
- Inflammatory cytokines can cause thrombocytopenia by destroying progenitors in the bone marrow and reducing platelet production.
- Finally, thrombocytopenia may be due to the presence of autoantibodies, and the destruction of platelets. Case studies of patients developing idiopathic thrombocytopenia purpura (ITP) and thrombotic thrombocytopenic purpura (TTP) following SARS-CoV-2 infection have been published with the likely mechanism being the molecular mimicry between the antigens of SARS-CoV-2 and platelet glycoproteins.

EFFECT ON BONE MARROW

Hemophagocytosis has been found in the bone marrow aspirates of severe COVID-19 patients with an increase in pleomorphic megakaryocytes, plasma cells, and macrophages. Rare virions were also identified in bone marrow megakaryocytes using electron microscopy.[11] Direct viral effects on the hematopoietic stem cells may affect hematopoiesis.

COAGULOPATHY IN COVID-19

The imbalance between coagulation and fibrinolysis in the pulmonary circulation and bronchoalveolar space are likely to be important factors in the pathogenesis of ARDS in COVID-19.

- Elevated D-dimer levels (>1,000 ng/mL), decreased fibrinogen (<1.0 g/L) and increased prothrombin times were seen in COVID-19.[12] Thrombotic complications include pulmonary embolism, venous thromboembolic events such as proximal deep vein and upper extremity thrombosis, and arterial thromboembolic events such as ischemic strokes were seen in around 25–31% of intensive care unit (ICU) admitted COVID-19.
- Bleeding is uncommon in the COVID-19 patients with DIC which is similar to the SARS-CoV-1 infection however rate of thrombosis is three to six times higher.[13]
- COVID-19 patients admitted to the ICU may have other risk factors (such as old age, obesity, and smoking) that may aggravate coagulopathy. Patients with co-morbid conditions (e.g. disease, obesity); a SIC (sepsis-induced coagulopathy) score ≥4 and elevated levels of D-dimer (>6 times ULN), C-reactive protein, troponins; and other markers of disseminated intravascular coagulopathy (DIC) are associated with a worse prognosis.[14]

Treatment

- The routine use of antithrombotic prophylaxis with low-molecular-weight heparin is recommended for inpatients by the International Society on Thrombosis and Hemostasis given the relatively high rates of VTE. LMWH has advantages over UFH with once-daily versus twice or thrice daily injections and less heparin-induced thrombocytopenia. However, they are contraindicated in ESRD, active bleeding, platelets <20,000/mm³, and BP >200/120 mm Hg.[9]
- Direct oral anti-coagulants DOACs (Rivaroxaban, Apixaban) are approved for in-hospital prophylaxis, however, these agents should be considered with caution in COVID-19 patients in whom coadministration of immunosuppressant, anti-viral, and other experimental therapies may hamper with DOAC therapeutic activity.

Anticoagulants	Doses
Inj. Enoxaparin	40 mg SC OD Contraindicated in ESRD
Inj. UFH	5000 SC BD in ESRD
Apixaban	2.5 mg BD
Rivaroxaban	10 mg OD Avoid use in CrCL <15 ml/min
Dabigatran	5–10 days of parental therapy with 150 mg BD Not recommended if CrCL <30 ml/min

Duration of Anti-coagulation

- In the absence of COVID-19 specific data, the rationale behind extended duration thromboprophylaxis with LMWH or a DOAC for at least 2 weeks is due to high rates of VTE observed in patients.

- Prolonged anti-coagulation is recommended for 6 weeks post-hospital discharge in selected COVID-19 patients with significant VTE risk factors such as advanced age, stay in the ICU, cancer, a prior history of VTE, thrombophilia, severe immobility, an elevated D-dimer (>2 times ULN), and an IMPROVE VTE score of 4 or more and who are at low-risk of bleeding.
- In the case of confirmed VTE, the duration of treatment should be at least 3 months.[14]

COVID-19 IN HEMATOLOGICAL DISORDERS

In bleeding disorders, the COVID-19 clinical manifestations were similar to other patients.[15] As hematologic malignancies directly affect the immune system, these patients are at significantly higher risk of a variety of severe infections including COVID-19. Therapeutic side effects such as myelosuppression and lymphodepletion and direct immunosuppression may make such patients more prone to infections. Patients with hematologic, lung, or metastatic (stage IV) cancer had more severe disease and higher mortality than those without malignancy.[16]

It is important to individually evaluate the necessity of active intervention, postponing elective surgery or adjuvant chemotherapy for patients with low-risk of progression, and minimising outpatient visits for mitigating exposure and transmission.

VACCINATION IN COVID-19

COVID-19 vaccination campaigns with several vaccine types are currently underway worldwide to combat COVID-19. The vaccines that have been developed are highly effective with minimal adverse effects. Currently, AstraZeneca and Covaxin vaccines have been approved to be administered to the Indian population and they are given as an intramuscular injection.

- Individuals receiving direct oral anticoagulant (apixaban, dabigatran, edoxaban and rivaroxaban) or warfarin in therapeutic INR range or on full-dose heparin or fondaparinux injections can all receive the COVID-19 vaccination. It is recommended to apply prolonged pressure (at least 5 minutes) to the injection site after vaccination to reduce bruising. Patients taking warfarin with supra-therapeutic INR should delay vaccination until their INR is <3.
- Patients with low platelet disorders like ITP, platelet function disorders (like Glanzmann thrombasthenia, Hermansky Pudlak syndrome, Grey Platelet syndrome), or platelet disorders caused by medications (such as aspirin, clopidogrel, ticagrelor) should take extra precautions when receiving the vaccine to prevent hematoma formation. A fine-gauge needle (25 or 27 gauge) should be used for the vaccination, followed by pressure on the site, without rubbing, for at least 10 minutes. Platelet count should not be less than 50,000/mm^3.[17]
- Patients with hemophilia should get a prior dose of factor concentrates before vaccination.
- Vaccination can be administered to patients with malignancies including hematological malignancies with a prior complete blood count profile.
- Vaccine-induced immune thrombotic thrombocytopenia: Recently, the Astra Zeneca vaccine and Johnson and Johnson (J and J) vaccine, both of them adenoviral vector-

based vaccines have raised a public alarm with concerns regarding the rare, but serious, development of thrombotic events such as cerebral sinus vein and splanchnic vein thrombosis, now known as vaccine-induced immune thrombotic thrombo-cytopenia (VIITT). These thrombotic events appear similar to heparin-induced thrombocytopenia, both clinically and pathologically with the presence of high-titer anti-PF4/heparin antibodies that cause platelet activation in functional assays. The risk of developing the HIT-like clotting syndrome is very low, with 86 potential cases reported in Europe out of 25 million people vaccinated as of 22 March.[18]

VIITT is treated with high dose IVIg and non-heparin anticoagulation after high clinical suspicion and positive laboratory parameters.[19]

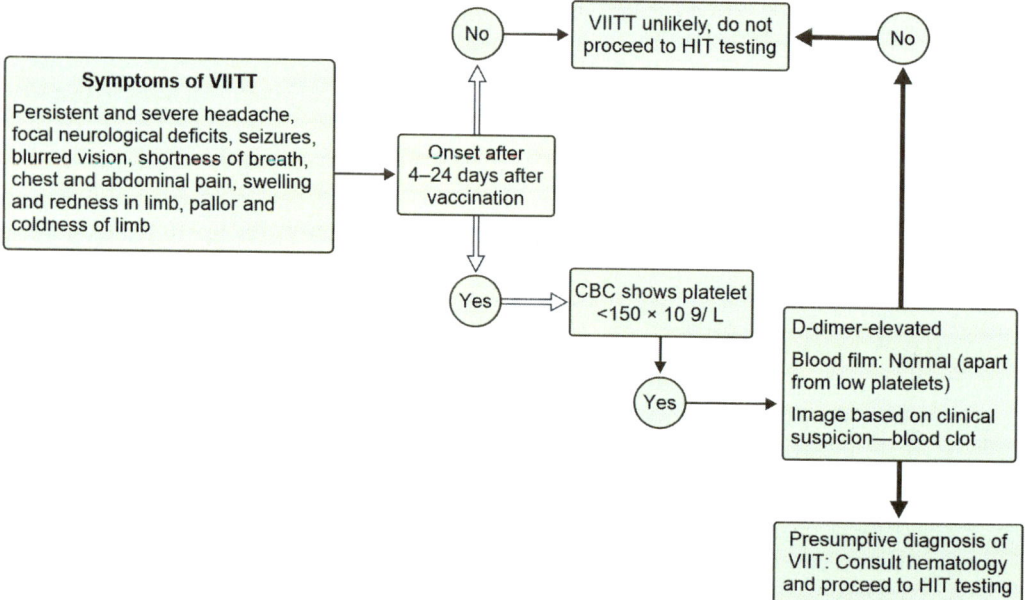

Conclusion

Lymphocytopenia, thrombocytopenia, and increased D-dimer are common hematological abnormalities in COVID-19 and are utilized for both diagnosis and prognosis. Attention needs to be paid to coagulation abnormalities and steps taken to prevent the complications related to it.

Vaccines are efficacious and safe against COVID-19, thereby they can be administered to all individuals irrespective of underlying hematological condition with due precautions.

REFERENCES

1. Coronavirus disease (COVID-19)–World Health Organization [Internet]. Available from: https://www.who.int/emergencies/diseases/novel-coronavirus-2019.
2. Amiral J, Vissac AM, Seghatchian J. COVID-19, induced activation of hemostasis, and immune reactions: Can an auto-immune reaction contribute to the delayed severe complications observed in some patients? Transfus Apher Sci Off J World Apher Assoc Off J Eur Soc Haemapheresis. 2020 Jun; 59(3):102–804.

3. Ulrich H, Pillat MM. CD147 as a Target for COVID-19 Treatment: Suggested Effects of Azithromycin and Stem Cell Engagement. Stem Cell Rev Rep. 2020 Jun; 16(3):434–40.

4. Evidence for structural protein damage and membrane lipid remodeling in red blood cells from COVID-19 patients | medRxiv. Available from: https://www.medrxiv.org/content/10.1101/2020.06.29.20142703v1

5. Schapkaitz E, De Jager T, Levy B. The characteristic peripheral blood morphological features of hospitalized patients infected with COVID-19. Int J Lab Hematol. 2021 Jun; 43(3):e130–4.

6. Zhao Q, Meng M, Kumar R, Wu Y, Huang J, Deng Y, et al. Lymphopenia is associated with severe coronavirus disease 2019 (COVID-19) infections: A systemic review and meta-analysis. Int J Infect Dis. 2020 Jul; 96:131–5.

7. Karimi Shahri M, Niazkar HR, Rad F. COVID-19 and hematology findings based on the current evidences: A puzzle with many missing pieces. Int J Lab Hematol. 2021 Apr; 43(2):160–8.

8. Neutrophil-to-lymphocyte ratio as an independent risk factor for mortality in hospitalized patients with COVID-19–PubMed. Available from: https://pubmed.ncbi.nlm.nih.gov/32283162/

9. Clinical Management Protocol for COVID-19 dated 27062020.pdf [Internet]. [cited 2021 Jul 15]. Available from: https://www.mohfw.gov.in/pdf/Clinical Management Protocol for COVID-19 dated27062020.pdf

10. Rahman A, Niloofa R, Jayarajah U, De Mel S, Abeysuriya V, Seneviratne SL. Hematological Abnormalities in COVID-19: A Narrative Review. Am J Trop Med Hyg. 2021 Feb 19; tpmd201536.

11. Debliquis A, Harzallah I, Mootien J, Poidevin A, Guylaine L, Mejri A, et al. Haemophagocytosis in bone marrow aspirates in patients with COVID-19. Br J Haematol. 2020 Jun 12;190.

12. COVID-19 and coagulopathy—Hematology.org. Available from: https://www.hematology.org:443/covid-19/covid-19-and-coagulopathy

13. Iba T, Levy JH, Levi M, Thachil J. Coagulopathy in COVID19. J Thromb Haemost. 2020 Jun 18;10.1111/jth.14975.

14. Spyropoulos AC, Levy JH, Ageno W, Connors JM, Hunt BJ, Iba T, et al. Scientific and Standardization Committee communication: Clinical guidance on the diagnosis, prevention, and treatment of venous thromboembolism in hospitalized patients with COVID-19. J Thromb Haemost. 2020; 18(8):1859–65.

15. Clinical findings in a patient with haemophilia A affected by COVID-19 - PubMed [Internet]. [cited 2021 Jul 15]. Available from: https://pubmed.ncbi.nlm.nih.gov/32239590/

16. COVID-19 in persons with haematological cancers | Leukemia [Internet]. Available from: https://www.nature.com/articles/s41375-020-0836-7

17. COVID-19 Vaccine FAQs [Internet]. Available from: https://www.mohfw.gov.in/covid_vaccination/vaccination/faqs.html

18. Ledford H. How could a COVID vaccine cause blood clots? Scientists race to investigate. Nature. 2021 Apr; 592(7854):334–5.

19. Nazy I, Sachs UJ, Arnold DM, McKenzie SE, Choi P, Althaus K, et al. Recommendations for the clinical and laboratory diagnosis of VITT against COVID-19: Communication from the ISTH SSC Subcommittee on Platelet Immunology. J Thromb Haemost. 2021; 19(6):1585–8.

Bibliography

1. (COVID-19) infection and pregnancy. Guidance for Healthcare professionals on coronavirus (COVID-19) infection in pregnancy, published by the RCOG, Royal College of Midwives, Royal College of Paediatrics and Child Health, Public Health England and Health Protection Scotland. Version 4.1. Updated 26 March, 2020.

2. Ai JW, ZhangY, Zhang HC, et al. Era ofmolecular diagnosis for pathogen identification of unexplained pneumonia, lessons to be learned. Emerg Microbes Infect. 2020;9(1):597–600.

3. Ai T, Yang Z, Hou H, et al. Correlation ofchest CT and RT-PCR testing in coronavirus disease 2019 (COVID-19) in China: A report of 1014 cases. Radiology. Available at: https://pubs.rsna.org/doi/ 10.1148/radiol.2020200642. Accessed Mar 16, 2020.

4. Akalin E, Azzi Y, Bartash R, et al. Covid-19 and kidney transplantation. N Engl J Med. 2020; NEJMe2011117. [Epub ahead of print]

5. Alanagreh L, Alzoughool F, Atoum M. The human coronavirus disease COVID-19: Its origin, characteristics, and insights into potential drugs and its mechanisms. Pathogens. 2020,905):331.

6. Alhazzani W, Moller MH, Arabi YM, et al. Surviving Sepsis Campaign: guidelines on the management of critically ill adults with coronavirus disease 2019(COVID-19). Intensive Care Med. 2020;46(5):854–87.

7. Andrews G, Basu A, CuijpersP, et al. Computer therapy for the anxiety and depression disorders is effective, acceptable and practical health care: An updated meta-analysis. J Anxiety Disord. 2018;55:70–8.

8. Arkin A, Krishnan K, Chang MG, et al. Nutrition in critically ill patients with COVID-19: challenges and special considerations. Clin Nutr. 2020;39(7):2327–8.

9. Available at: https://www.mohfw.gov.in/pdf/PreventivemeasuresDOPT.pdf

10. Available at: www.worldometer.info/coronavirus.

11. Bauch CT, Lloyd-Smith JO, Coffee MP, et al. Dynamically modeling SARS and other newly emerging respiratory illnesses: past, present, and future. Epidemiology. 2005; 16(6):791–801.

12. Bayliss DA, Millhorn DE. Central neural mechanisms of progesterone action: application to the respiratory system. J Appl Physiol. 1992;73(2):393–404.

13. Bhatraju PK, Ghassemieh BJ, Nichols M, et al. Covid-19 in critically ill patients in the Seattle region–case series. N Engl J Med. 2020;382(21):2012–22.

14. Bhattacharya N, Bhattacharya K. Informed consent for surgery during COVID-19. Indian J Surg. 2020;1-3. [Epubhed of print].

15. Brooks SK, Webster RK, Smith LE, et al. The psychological impact of quarantine and how to reduce it: rapid review of the evidence. Lancet Lond Engl. 2020;395(10227):912.

16. Cascella M, Rajnik M, Cuomo A, et al. Features, evaluation and treatment coronavirus (COVID-19). [Updated 2020 Mar 20]. In: StatPearls [Internet]. Treasure Island (FL): StatPearls Publishing; 2020 Jan-. Available from: https://www.ncbi.nlm.nih.gov/books/ NBK554776/

17. CDC. Considerations for inpatient obstetric healthcare settings care for pregnant women. Updated May 20, 2020. Available at: https://www.cdc.gov/coronavirus/2019 ncov/hcp/inpatient-obstetric-healthcare-guidance.html

18. Cheng Y, Luo R, Wang K, et al. Kidney disease is associated with in-hospital death of patients with COVID-19. Kidney Int. 2020;97(5):829–38.

19. Coccolini F, Perrone G, Chiarugi M, et al. Surgery in COVID-19 patients: operational directives. World J Emerg Surg. 2020; 15 (1):25.

20. Connors JM, Levy JH. Thromboinflammation and the hypercoagulability of COVID-19.JThrombHaemost. 202018(7):1559–61.

21. Corman VM, Landt 0, Kaiser M, et al. Detection of 2019 novel coronavirus (2019-nCoV) by real-time RT-PCR. Euro Surveill. 2020;25(3):2000045.

22. Coronavirus (COVID-19), pregnancy, and breastfeeding: a message for patients. Available at: https://www. acog.org/patient-resources/faqs/pregnancy/coronaviruspregnancy-and-breastfeeding

23. Coronavirus Perinatal–Neonatal management of COVID-19 Infection, Clinical Practice Guidelines, FOGSI. Ver. 2.0. May 2020.

24. COVID-19. Indian Council of Medical Research, Government of India. Available at:https://www.icmr.nic.in/content/covid-19. Accessed Mar 16, 2020.

25. Diao B, Wen K, Chen J, et al. Diagnosis of acute respiratory syndrome coronavirus 2 infection by detection of nucleocapsid protein. medRxi 2020.03.07.20032524. Available at: https://www.medrxiv.org/content/10.1101/2020.03.07.200325242. Accessed Apr 12, 2020.

26. Elshafeey F, Magdi R, Hindi N, et al. A systematic scoping review of COVID-19 during pregnancy and childbirth. Int J Gynaecol Obstet. 2020;150(1):47–52.

27. Grasselli G, Zangrillo A, Zanella A, et al. Baseline characteristics and outcomes of 1591 patients infected with SARS-CoV-2 admitted to ICUs of the Lombardy region, Italy. JAMA. 2020;323(16):1574–81.

28. Guan WJ, Ni ZY, Hu Y, et al. Clinical characteristics of coronavirus disease 2019 in China. N Engl J Med. 2020;382(18):1708–20.

29. Hantoushzadeh S, Shamshirsaz AA, Aleyasin A, et al. Maternal death due to COVID-19. Am J Obstet Gynecol. 2020;223(1):109.e1–109.e16.

30. Henry BM, Lippi G. Chronic kidney disease is associated with severe coronavirus disease 2019 (COVID-19) infection. Int UrolNephrol. 2020;52(6):1193–4.

31. Hopman J, Allegranzi B, Mehtar S. Managing COVID-19 in low- and middle-income countries. JAMA. 2020;323(16):1549–50.

32. http://isnindia.org/UserFiles/Image/COVID 19%20working%20group%20of%20 ISN%20 India.pdf

33. https://coronavirus.jhu.edu/map.html

34. https://www.mohfw.gov.in/pdf RevisedguidelinesforHomeisolationofverymildpre-symptomaticCOVID 19c ases 10May2020.pdf

35. https://www.mohfw.gov.in/pdf/ReviseddischargePolicyforCOVID19.pdf

36. Huang C, Wang Y, Li X, et al. Clinical features of patients infected with 2019 novel coronavirus in Wuhan, China. Lancet. 2020;395(10223):497–506.

37. Hui OS, Chan MT, Chow B. Aerosol dispersion during various respiratory therapies: a risk assessment model of nosocomial infection to health care workers. Hong Kong Med J. 2014;20 Suppl 4:9–13.

38. Human coronavirus types. CDC. Available at: https://www.cdc.gov/ coronavirus/types. html

39. Inter association surgical practice recommendations in Covid 19 era (For minimal access surgeons). Available from www.amasi.org.

40. Kaushik S, Kaushik S, Sharma Y, et al. The Indian perspective of COVID-19 outbreak, VirusDis. 2020;1–8.

41. Laboratory testing for 2019 novel coronavirus (2019-nCoV) in suspected human cases. WHO, 19 March, 2020. Available at: https://www.who.int/publications-detail/ laboratory-testing-for-2019-novel-coronavirus-in-suspected-human-cases-20200117. Accessed Mar 15, 2020.

42. Lei S, Jiang F, Su W, et al. Clinical characteristics and outcomes of patients undergoing surgeries during the incubation period of COVID-19 infection. E Clin Med. 2020;21: 100331.

43. Li J, FinkJB, Ehrmann S. High-flow nasal cannula for COVID-19 patients: low risk of bio-aerosol dispersion. Eur Respir J. 2020;20(5):2000892.

44. Li Q, Guan X, Wu P, et al. Early transmission dynamics in Wuhan, China, of novel coronavirus-infected pneumonia. N Engl J Med. 2020;382(13):1199–207.

45. Li X, Geng M, Peng Y, et al. Molecular immune pathogenesis and diagnosis of COVID-19.J Pharm Anal. 2020;10(2):102–8.

46. Liao X, Wang B, Kang Y. Novel coronavirus infection during the 2019-2020 epidemic: preparing intensive care units—the experience in Sichuan Province, China. Intensive Care Med. 2020;4602):357–60.

47. Liu J, Liao X, Qian S, et al. Community transmission of severe acute respiratory syndrome coronavirus 2, Shenzhen, China, 2020. Emerg Infect Dis. 2020;26(6):1320–3.

48. Malhotra N, Joshi M, Datta R, et al. Indian Society of Anaesthesiologists (ISA National) Advisory and Position Statement regarding COVID-19. Indian J Anaesth. 2020;64(4):259–63.

49. Mancia G, Rea F, LudergnaniM, et al. Renin-angiotensin-aldosterone system blockers and the risk ofCovid-19.N Engl J Med. 2020;NEJMoa2006923. [Epub ahead ofprint]

50. Manuell ME, Cukor J. Mother nature versus human nature: public compliance with evacuation and quarantine. Disasters. 2011;35(2):417–42.

51. Masters PS. The molecular biology of coronaviruses. Acv Virus Res. 2006;66:193–292.

52. Morris SN, Fader AN, Milad MP, et al. Understanding the "Scope" of the problem: Why laparoscopy is considered safe during the COVID-19 pandemic. J Minim Invasive Gynecol. 2020;27(4):789–91.

53. Mullins PM, Goyal M, Pines JM. National growth in intensive care unit admissions from emer-gency departments in the United States from 2002 to 2009. AcadEmerg Med. 2013;20(5): 479–86.

54. Ong SWX, Tan YK, Chia PY, et al. Air, surface environmental, and personal protective equipment contamination by severe acute respiratory syndrome coronavirus 2 (SARSCoV-2) from a symptomatic patient. JAMA. 2020;323(16):1610–2.

55. Packaging and Shipping Clinical Specimens Diagram I For Laboratory Personnel. Ebola (Ebola Virus Disease). CDC. 2019. Available at: https://www.cdc.gov/vhf/ebola/laboratory-personnel/shipping-specimens.html. Accessed Apr 11, 2020.

56. Phua J, Weng L, Ling L, et al. 2019(C0OVID-19): challenges 2020,8(5):506–17. Intensive care management of coronavirus disease and recommendations. Lancet Respir Med.

57. Psychiatry of Pandemics] SpringerLink [Internet]. [cited 2020 Aug 11]. Available from: https://link.springer.com/book/10.1007%2F978-3-030-15346-5

58. Quarantine and Isolation I Quarantine I CDC [Internet]. 2019 [cited 2020 Aug 11]. Available from: https://www.cdc.gov/quarantine/index.html

59. RazaiMS, Oakeshott P, Kankam H, et al. Mitigating the psychological effects of social isolation during the covid-19 pandemic. BM] 2020;369:m1904.

60. Ren LL, Wang YM, Wu ZQ, et al. Identification of a novel corona virus causing severe pneumonia in human: a descriptive study. Chin Med J (Engl). 2020; 133(9):1015–24.

61. Ren LL, Wang YM, Wu ZQ, et al. Identification of a novel coronavirus causing severe pneumonia in human: a descriptive study. Chin Med J (Engl). 2020;133(9):1015–24.

62. Revised Guidelines on Clinical Management of COVID-19. Government of India, Ministry of Health and Family Welfare, Directorate General of Health Services (EMR Division). 31st March, 2020. Available at: https://www.mohfw.gov.in/pdf/RevisedNationalClinicalManagement GuidelineforCOVID1931032020.pdf.

63. Richardson S, Hirsch JS, Narasimhan M, et al. Presenting characteristics, comorbidities, and outcomes among 5700 patients hospitalized with COVID-19 in the New York City area. JAMA. 2020;323(20):2052–9.

64. SARS-CoV-2 variants (who.int).new added

65. Snijder EJ, van der Meer Y, Zevenhoven-Dobbe J, et al. Ultrastructure and origin of membrane vesicles associated with the severe acute respiratory syndrome coronavirus replication complex. J Virol. 2006;80(12):5927–40.

66. Social Consequences of Ebola Containment Measures in Liberia [Internet]. [cited 2020 Aug 1H]. Available from: https://journals.plos.org/plosone/article?id=10.1371/journal. pone.0143036

67. Social prescribing. BMJ. 2019;364:11285. Available at: https://www.bmj.com/content/364/bmj.l11285

68. Spoorthy MS, Pratapa SK, Mahant S. Mental health problems faced by healthcare workers due to the COVID-19 pandemic - A review. Asian J Psychiatry. 2020;51:102119

69. Su H, Yang M, Wan C, et al. Renal histopathological analysis of26 postmortem findings of patients with COVID-19 in China. Kidney Int. 2020;$0085-2538(20)30369-0. [Epub ahead of print]

70. Understanding, compliance and psychological impact ofthe SARS quarantine experience I Epidemiology and Infection I Cambridge Core [Internet]. [cited 2020 Aug 11]. Available from: https://www.cambridge.org/core/journals/epidemiology-and-infection/article/understanding-compliance-and-psychological-impact-of-the-sars-quarantine-experienc e/7AE55E5054DEC1A1D23679FD9E05A52B

71. W~lfelR, Corman VM, Guggemos W, et al. Virological assessment of hospitalized patients with COVID-2019. Nature. 2020;581(7809):465–9.

72. Wang SF, Chen KH, Chen M, et al. Human-leukocyte antigen class ICw 1502 and class II DR 0301 genotypes are associated with resistance to severe acute respiratory syndrome (SARS) infection. Viral Immunol. 2011;24(5):421–6.

73. Wang W, Xu Y, Gao R, et al. Detection of SARS-CoV-2 in different types of clinical specimens. JAMA. 2020;323(18):1843–4.

74. Wei M, Yuan J, Liu Y, et al. Novel coronavirus infection in hospitalized infants under 1 year of age in China. JAMA. 2020;323(13):1313–4.

75. Wei WE, Li Z, Chiew CJ, et al. Presymptomatic transmission of SARS CoV-2—Singapore, January 23—March 16, 2020. MMWR Morb Mortal Wkly Rep. 2020;69:411–5.

76. Wester M, Giesecke J. Ebola and healthcare worker stigma. Scand J Public Health. 2019;47(2):99–04.

77. Whittle JS, Pavlov I, SacchettiAD, et al. Respiratory support for adult patients with COVID-19. JACEP Open. 2020;1–7.

78. WHO. Coronavirus disease (COVID-19) advice for the public. Available at: https://www.who.int/emergencies/diseases/novel-coronavirus-2019/advice-for-public

79. Why do we need antibody tests for COVID-19 and how to interpret test results. In: Diazyme Laboratories. Available at: http://www.diazyme.com/covid-19-antibody-tests. Accessed Apr 13, 2020.

80. World Health Organization. Mental health and psychosocial considerations during the COVID-19 outbreak. 2020. Available at: https://www.who.int/docs/default-source/coronaviruse/mental-health-considerations pdf.

81. World Health Organization. Report of the WHO-China Joint Mission on Coronavirus Disease 2019 (COVID-19). 16-24 February, 2020 [Internet]. Geneva: World Health Organization; 2020. Available at: https://www.who. int/docs/default-source/coronaviruse/who-china-joint-mission-on-covid19-finalreport.pdf

82. Wu Z, McGoogan JM. Characteristics of and important lessons from the coronavirus disease 2019 (COVID-19) outbreak in China: Summary of a report of 72 314 cases from the Chinese Center for Disease Control and Prevention. JAMA. 2020;10.1001/ jama.2020.2648. [Epub ahead of print]

83. Xiao F, Tang M, Zheng X, et al. Evidence for gastrointestinal infection of SARS-CoV-2. Gastroenterology. 2020;158:1831–3.

84. XiongF, Tang H, Liu L, et al. Clinical characteristics of and medical interventions for COVID-19 in hemodialysis patients in Wuhan, China. J Am Soc Nephrol. 2020;ASN.2020030354. [Epub ahead of print]

85. Zhang Y, Chen C, Zhu S, et al. Isolation of 2019-nCoV from a stool specimen of a laboratory-confirmed case of the coronavirus disease 2019 (COVID-19). China CDC Weekly. 2020;2(8):123–4.

86. Zhou P, Yang XL, Wang XG, et al. A pneumonia outbreak associated with a new coronavirus of probable bat origin. Nature. 2020;579(7798):270–3.

87. Zou L, Ruan F, Huang M, et al. SARS-CoV-2 viral load in upper respiratory specimens of infected patients. N Engl J Med. 2020;382(12):1177–9.

Index